A PATIENT'S GUIDE TO CANCER SYMPTOM MANAGEMENT

by Carlton G. Brown, PhD, RN, AOCN®

Hygeia Media
An imprint of the Oncology Nursing Society
Pittsburgh, Pennsylvania

ONS Publications Department
Interim Publisher and Director of Publications: Barbara Sigler, RN, MNEd
Managing Editor: Lisa M. George, BA
Technical Content Editor: Angela D. Klimaszewski, RN, MSN
Staff Editor II: Amy Nicoletti, BA
Copy Editor: Laura Pinchot, BA
Graphic Designer: Dany Sjoen

Library of Congress Cataloging-in-Publication Data

Brown, Carlton G. (Carlton Gene)
A patient's guide to cancer symptom management / by Carlton G Brown.
p. cm.
ISBN 978-1-935864-01-1 (alk. paper)
1. Cancer--Treatment--Popular works. 2. Cancer--Psychological aspects--Popular works. I. Title.
RC263.B72 2010
616.99'4--dc22

2010045621

Publisher's Note

This book is published by the Oncology Nursing Society (ONS). ONS neither represents nor guarantees that the practices described herein will, if followed, ensure safe and effective patient care. The recommendations contained in this book reflect ONS's judgment regarding the state of general knowledge and practice in the field as of the date of publication. The recommendations may not be appropriate for use in all circumstances. Those who use this book should make their own determinations regarding specific safe and appropriate patient-care practices, taking into account the personnel, equipment, and practices available at the hospital or other facility at which they are located. The author and publisher cannot be held responsible for any liability incurred as a consequence from the use or application of any of the contents of this book. Figures and tables are used as examples only. They are not meant to be all-inclusive, nor do they represent endorsement of any particular institution by ONS. Mention of specific products and opinions related to those products do not indicate or imply endorsement by ONS. Web sites mentioned are provided for information only; the hosts are responsible for their own content and availability. Unless otherwise indicated, dollar amounts reflect U.S. dollars.

ONS publications are originally published in English. Publishers wishing to translate ONS publications must contact ONS about licensing arrangements. ONS publications cannot be translated without obtaining written permission from ONS. (Individual tables and figures that are reprinted or adapted require additional permission from the original source.) Because translations from English may not always be accurate or precise, ONS disclaims any responsibility for inaccuracies in words or meaning that may occur as a result of the translation. Readers relying on precise information should check the original English version.

Printed in the United States of America

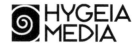

An imprint of the Oncology Nursing Society

I would like to dedicate this book to my father, Harold Gene Brown, for his own personal fight against the disease and adverse symptoms that I have ironically worked my entire adult life to eradicate.

And to all the patients with cancer who have touched my life along the way and who remind me every day that my service as an oncology nurse is important.

Contents

Preface

I F YOU ARE READING THIS BOOK, YOU OR SOMEONE you know has probably been diagnosed with cancer. This book was written with the patient and family in mind because I realized early on that many books and information are available to help healthcare providers care for patients with cancer, but very little information is available for the actual patient and family. It is my hope that this book will fill that void and perhaps will help you or someone you know understand and better manage the symptoms sometimes associated with cancer and treatment.

I firmly believe in the adage that "knowledge is power." For patients starting cancer treatment, prior knowledge about possible symptoms that they may experience better prepares them to know what to do when they experience these symptoms. As a cancer nurse working with patients and families for the past 20 years, I have seen firsthand how symptoms, especially those that go unattended, can have an overall effect in the course of cancer treatment. When symptoms are managed, patients have better outcomes. On the other hand, when patients have symptoms such as nausea and vomiting that go untreated, the experience can be dreadful. I have witnessed patients who had symptoms so severe that they sometimes requested to stop or decrease treatment. This is unfortunate because almost all of the symptoms discussed in this book can be treated. When patients learn that they will receive some sort of cancer treatment, such as chemotherapy or radiation, the first questions they often ask are

- Will I lose my hair?
- Will I have nausea and vomiting?
- Will I be in pain?

These are all symptoms, in addition to many others, that are addressed in this book.

As I have mentioned, this book was written with the patient in mind. Plain language is used instead of medical jargon so that potentially everyone who reads it will hopefully understand it. I have learned that during these very difficult times, the easier the material is to understand, the more likely it is to be remembered and applied. You will also notice that the book is focused by presenting common questions that patients have, followed by answers that are factual and based in as much evidence as possible.

Finally, this book can be read from beginning to end in a very short period of time for general knowledge of the major symptoms that patients sometimes experience. Perhaps more importantly, this book can be referred to when the patient begins to experience any symptom, such as hair loss, nausea, or pain.

It is my hope that you will find this book useful and helpful. It is not intended to replace conversations with your doctor or another healthcare provider but rather to help you be better informed about the symptoms you or someone you care for might experience. During this challenging time, I wish you a high-quality experience, free of as many symptoms as possible. If by chance you do experience symptoms, I hope you or someone you care for finds this book helpful in alleviating those symptoms so that you can gain the most benefit from your cancer treatment.

Acknowledgments

I would like to extend a special thanks to Barbara Sigler for her support in this book and helping the idea become reality and to Eleanor Mayfield, ELS, for her editorial assistance with the preparation of this book.

CHAPTER 1

Anemia

What Is Anemia?

A NEMIA IS A SHORTAGE OF RED BLOOD CELLS AND of hemoglobin, a substance in red blood cells whose job is to carry oxygen around the body. Without hemoglobin, no oxygen is delivered to the cells. Just as you need oxygen to breathe, your body's cells need oxygen to function properly. A shortage of oxygen can have a wide variety of effects on almost every part of your body. Anemia is a very common problem in people with cancer, especially those who are being treated with chemotherapy or radiation. Some patients have anemia before they even begin treatment, which makes the overall problem even more difficult.

What Causes Anemia in People With Cancer?

Anemia in people with cancer can have a number of different causes. What these causes have in common is that they interfere with the body's ability to make new red blood cells. A shortage of red blood cells means a shortage of hemoglobin to carry the oxygen your body needs.

Normally, your kidneys produce a hormone called erythropoietin (eh-RITH-roh-POY-eh-tin) that stimulates the bone marrow to make red blood cells. One of the effects of cancer can be to slow down the kidneys' ability to make this hormone. With less erythropoietin being made, the bone marrow does not get the stimulus it needs to make a normal number of new red blood cells.

Patients who receive chemotherapy with drugs that contain platinum (for example, carboplatin, cisplatin, or oxaliplatin) have an especially high risk for anemia because these drugs can damage the kidneys. Damaged kidneys produce less erythropoietin. As a result, the bone marrow gets less of a stimulus to make new red blood cells, so it produces fewer of them.

People with cancer can also get anemia in other ways.

- Chemotherapy or radiation can cause anemia by damaging the bone marrow. Damaged bone marrow makes fewer red blood cells than healthy bone marrow.
- Normal red blood cells live about 120 days, and then die.
- In people with cancer, red blood cells wear out faster than they do in healthy people. When red blood cells die more quickly than the body can replace them, pretty soon the body has a shortage of red blood cells.
- Having too little iron in the blood can cause anemia. Without enough iron, the blood cannot make enough hemoglobin to carry oxygen around the body.
- Losing a lot of blood through surgery or internal bleeding may cause anemia.
- Patients with cancer who are not eating well can get anemia because their diet lacks essential nutrients, especially iron.

What Are the Symptoms of Anemia?

The most common symptoms of anemia are feeling tired, difficulty breathing (shortness of breath), and low energy.

However, mild anemia may have no symptoms or very few obvious symptoms.

Having a low red blood cell count or hemoglobin count means your body is not getting enough oxygen. A shortage of oxygen can affect your body in many different ways (see Symptoms of Anemia).

Symptoms of Anemia

In addition to tiredness, difficulty breathing (shortness of breath), and lack of energy, symptoms of anemia may include

- Apathy
- Cold skin
- Constipation
- Dizziness when moving from a lying to a standing position
- Dry or thinning hair
- Feeling irritable
- Headache
- Nails that break easily
- Pale skin
- Rapid heart beat
- Running a fever
- Sores in the mouth
- Swelling in the legs or feet
- Upset stomach

Can I Do Anything to Prevent Anemia?

If you have cancer, it is not easy to prevent anemia, but you may be able to prevent it from becoming serious. Tell a member of your healthcare team right away if you have any of the symptoms listed under Symptoms of Anemia. Treatment of cancer-related anemia may be more effective if it is started early, before symptoms become severe.

How Is Anemia Diagnosed?

Anemia is diagnosed with blood tests. These tests measure how much iron and how many red cells are in your blood, as well as how much hemoglobin is in the red blood cells.

Other blood tests measure levels of vitamin B_{12} and folate (another B vitamin). Adequate amounts of these vitamins help the body to produce red blood cells.

In addition to these blood tests, a member of your health-care team will ask you about how tired you feel and how being tired and low on energy is affecting your life.

How Are People With Cancer Treated for Anemia?

The two main types of treatment for anemia in people with cancer are blood transfusions and drugs that help the body make more red blood cells. Most people who take drugs to treat anemia need to take iron supplements as well.

Blood Transfusions

Your doctor may recommend a blood transfusion if your hemoglobin level is extremely low or your anemia symptoms are very severe. A blood transfusion raises your hemoglobin level quickly. This may help you feel better for a while.

Blood transfusions, however, also pose risks for people with cancer. For example, a few people get infections and others may get a serious reaction that makes it hard to breathe. Because of these risks, your doctor will monitor and weigh the need for blood transfusions, only giving you a transfusion when it is important.

Drugs

Two drugs are now approved in the United States to treat anemia in people with cancer who are receiving chemotherapy: Procrit®, also called epoetin alfa, and Aranesp®, also called darbepoetin alfa.

Remember erythropoietin, the hormone produced by the kidneys that stimulates the bone marrow to make red blood cells? Like erythropoietin, both Procrit and Aranesp work by helping the body make more red blood cells. You may hear them referred to as erythropoietin-stimulating agents (ESAs).

Both drugs are given as injections (shots) under the skin. It usually takes at least a couple of weeks for the drugs to start working. If the shots cause discomfort, try putting ice or a pain-relieving cream or lotion on the site prior to injection.

In studies, patients with cancer who took one of these drugs while receiving chemotherapy
• Had higher hemoglobin levels
• Needed fewer blood transfusions
• Felt better
• Had more energy for activities of daily life.

Similar to blood transfusions, however, these drugs pose risks. Some patients with cancer who take them get high blood pressure or blood clots.

Iron Supplements

Most patients who take Procrit or Aranesp also need to take iron pills or get iron injections to make sure that the body has an ample, steady supply of iron.

Some recent studies suggest that iron injections may work better than pills. Iron that is injected goes directly into the blood, where it gets to work right away helping to build new red blood cells.

Iron pills, on the other hand, have to be digested first, so it takes longer for them to get to work. Iron pills may also cause side effects such as pain in the abdomen, nausea, vomiting, and constipation. If you take iron pills, taking them with food helps to reduce the risk of these side effects. Tell a member of your healthcare team right away if you have pain in the abdomen or other side effects that may be caused by iron pills.

What Else Can I Do to Cope With Anemia During My Cancer Treatment?

These tips may help you cope with anemia during your cancer treatment.

- Save energy by choosing the most important things you need to do each day. You can also spread the things you do out over an entire day instead of doing them all at once.
- Take short naps (no more than an hour at a time) during the day.
- Get eight hours of sleep every night.
- Take a walk or get some other exercise every day. Some studies show that exercise helps with tiredness during cancer treatment.
- Eat a healthy diet and drink plenty of fluids. Talk with a member of your healthcare team about whether it would be helpful for you to eat foods that are high in protein (for example, meat, eggs, peanut butter) or high in iron (for example, leafy green vegetables, red meat, cooked beans).
- Keep a journal of your symptoms.

For More Information

For additional information about anemia, see the following resources.

American Cancer Society

- Anemia in People With Cancer: www.cancer.org/Treatment/ TreatmentsandSideEffects/PhysicalSideEffects/Anemia/ index?sitearea=MBC

American Society of Clinical Oncology (ASCO)

- What to Know: The ASCO and ASH Guideline on Epoetin and Darbepoetin Treatment for Adults With Cancer:

www.cancer.net/patient/ASCO%20Resources/What%20
to%20Know/What%20to%20Know%20PDFs/What_to_
Know_Epoetin_and_Darbepoetin_Treatment.pdf

National Anemia Action Council

- Anemia and Cancer: www.anemia.org/patients/information
  -handouts/cancer/?handout=cancer%2F
- Are Iron Injections Right for You?: www.anemia.org/
  patients/feature-articles/content.php?contentid=000403&
  sectionid=00015

National Cancer Institute

- Managing Chemotherapy Side Effects: Anemia: www.cancer.
  gov/cancertopics/chemo-side-effects/anemia

Anxiety

What Is Anxiety?

S IMPLY PUT, ANXIETY IS A REACTION TO SOMEthing you see as a threat. Another term for anxiety is *distress*. It is perfectly normal to sometimes feel distressed when you have cancer. Furthermore, every person's feelings are unique. When you are facing cancer, there is no right or wrong time to feel distressed. However, certain events in the cancer journey can especially cause anxiety (see Some Events That Can Cause Anxiety or Distress in People With Cancer).

Some Events That Can Cause Anxiety or Distress in People With Cancer

- Finding a worrying sign or symptom (for example, a breast lump)
- Going through tests to find out the cause of the symptom
- Being diagnosed with cancer
- Waiting for cancer treatment to begin
- Getting treatment and dealing with its side effects
- Changing to a different type of treatment
- Finishing treatment
- Going home after a hospital stay
- Before seeing the doctor for a cancer checkup
- Having a symptom that could mean the cancer has come back
- When treatment fails and the cancer comes back or spreads

What Are the Symptoms of Anxiety?

Anxiety can express itself through both your body and your mind (see Symptoms of Anxiety).

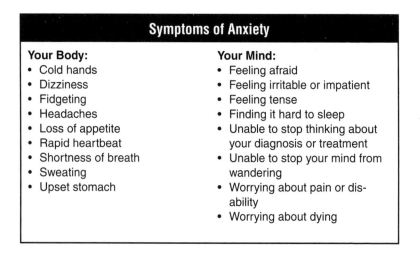

Symptoms of Anxiety

Your Body:
- Cold hands
- Dizziness
- Fidgeting
- Headaches
- Loss of appetite
- Rapid heartbeat
- Shortness of breath
- Sweating
- Upset stomach

Your Mind:
- Feeling afraid
- Feeling irritable or impatient
- Feeling tense
- Finding it hard to sleep
- Unable to stop thinking about your diagnosis or treatment
- Unable to stop your mind from wandering
- Worrying about pain or disability
- Worrying about dying

What Can I Do to Cope With Anxiety?

One of the best things you can do for yourself when you are feeling anxious or distressed is to talk about it. Studies show that talking about your fears can help to relieve them. Talk about your concerns with a member of your healthcare team. You may also wish to confide in a pastor, a family member, or a close friend.

Understanding your cancer, the plan for treating it, and how to manage your symptoms may also help you feel less distressed and more in control.

Many people who are facing cancer find it helpful to meet and talk with others facing the same diagnosis, sometimes referred to as a "buddy." Talk with a member of your healthcare team about joining a support group. Some support groups meet face to face and others interact by telephone or online. You may also want to consider individual counseling with a therapist or social worker who specializes in helping people with cancer.

Mind-body techniques may help to keep anxiety under control. These techniques include deep breathing, guided imagery (a systematic process of using your imagination to picture pleasant situations to help you to relax and relieve stress), meditation, yoga, and art or music therapy. Little or no research has been done to show whether these techniques are effective at relieving anxiety in people with cancer. Many individuals, however, find them helpful.

Pay attention to your feelings. Learn to identify the signs that you are becoming distressed or anxious. Try out some mind-body techniques. If you find one that helps you feel less anxious, use it when you feel yourself becoming distressed or before an event that makes you feel anxious.

Can Anxiety Be Treated With Medication?

If anxiety is seriously impairing your day-to-day life or your ability to go on with your cancer treatment, your doctor may prescribe a medication to treat it.

It is important to take the medication as directed and not to stop taking it without first talking to your doctor. Tell a member of your healthcare team if you feel dizzy or sleepy or if you notice other physical changes. These changes could be side effects of your medication for anxiety.

Medications for anxiety work best when they are combined with other coping strategies. So, take your medication, but keep on talking about your feelings, going to counseling or a support group, and using mind-body techniques that help relieve your distress.

For More Information

For additional information about anxiety, see the following resources.

American Cancer Society

- Anxiety Checklist for Patients: How Much Worry Is Normal When You Have Cancer?: www.cancer.org/Treatment/TreatmentsandSideEffects/EmotionalSideEffects/anxiety -checklist-for-patients?sitearea=MBC
- Anxiety, Fear, and Depression: www.cancer.org/Treatment/TreatmentsandSideEffects/EmotionalSideEffects/Anxiety FearandDepression/index?sitearea=MBC

American Society of Clinical Oncology

- Side Effects—Anxiety: www.cancer.net/patient/Coping/Emotional+and+Physical+Matters/Depression+and+Anxiety ?sectionTitle=Anxiety&sectionId=104466&vgnextrefresh=1

Oncology Nursing Society

- The Cancer Journey: Side Effects—Anxiety: www.thecancer journey.org/side/se-1

CHAPTER

Bone Loss and Osteoporosis

What Is the Link Between Bone Loss and Cancer Treatment?

W E MAY THINK OF OUR BONES AS SOLID AND unchanging. In fact, our bones are always changing. Throughout our lives, our bodies lose old bone and form new bone. We are in our peak bone-building years as children and teenagers. During this time, new bone formation outpaces the loss of old bone.

As we age, however, we start to lose old bone more quickly than our bodies can make new bone to replace it. Most women begin to lose bone mass at a faster pace around the time of the "change of life," or menopause. Men also lose bone mass as they age, but usually more slowly than women do.

As we lose bone mass, our bones become weaker and more likely to break. When bone loss becomes severe, it is known as osteoporosis (aw-stee-oh-puh-ROH-sis). Many people who have osteoporosis are not aware of it until they break a bone in their hip, spine, wrist, or elsewhere in the body.

Some types of cancer treatment can cause bone loss or make it worse (see Examples of Drugs Used in Cancer Treatment That May Result in Bone Loss). People with cancer who receive these treatments have an increased risk for bone loss that can lead to osteoporosis.

Examples of Drugs Used in Cancer Treatment That May Result in Bone Loss

Hormonal Therapies for Breast Cancer
- Anastrozole (Arimidex®)
- Exemestane (Aromasin®)
- Letrozole (Femara®)
- Tamoxifen (Nolvadex®)

Hormonal Therapies for Prostate Cancer
- Bicalutamide (Casodex®)
- Flutamide (Eulexin®)
- Goserelin (Zoladex®)
- Leuprolide (Lupron®)

Chemotherapy Drugs
- Dexamethasone (Decadron®)
- Ifosfamide (Ifex®)
- Methotrexate (Trexall®)
- Prednisone

What Are Hormonal Therapies and How Do They Cause Bone Loss?

Hormones are chemicals made by glands in the body. They circulate in the blood and control the actions of certain cells or organs. Among their other functions in the body, certain hormones (estrogen in women, testosterone in men) provide protection against bone loss.

Estrogen and testosterone can also, in some cases, play a role in helping cancer grow. Hormonal therapies are drugs that treat cancer by suppressing or blocking the body's ability to make or use these hormones. People with breast cancer or prostate cancer are treated with hormonal therapies.

If you are being treated with a hormonal therapy for cancer, your body may lack the protection against bone loss that estrogen or testosterone normally provides. Without this protection, you may have a higher risk for broken bones (fractures).

How Can Chemotherapy Cause Bone Loss?

Some chemotherapy drugs interfere with the body's ability to make new bone. Other drugs cause bone loss indirectly by disrupting the body's supply of estrogen or testosterone.

How Do I Know if I Have Bone Loss or Osteoporosis?

Bone loss happens silently and painlessly. There are no symptoms to alert you that your bones are getting weaker. A bone density scan, which is like an x-ray of the bones, is the only way to diagnose bone loss or osteoporosis. It is a painless test that measures the density of your bones. The most accurate type of bone density scan measures bone density in the hip and spine.

Talk with a member of your healthcare team about whether your cancer treatment will increase your risk for bone loss. If the answer is yes, ask if you should have a bone density scan.

What Can I Do to Prevent Bone Loss?

These steps can help you keep your bones healthy and reduce bone loss.

Consume plenty of calcium and vitamin D. Calcium helps keep bones strong. Vitamin D helps the body absorb calcium (see How Much Calcium and Vitamin D Do I Need? and Good

Dietary Sources of Calcium and Vitamin D). If you find it hard to eat enough foods that are high in calcium and vitamin D, it is fine to take supplements.

How Much Calcium and Vitamin D Do I Need?		
Age	**Calcium**	**Vitamin D**
Younger than age 50	1,000 mg per day	400–600 International Units (IU) per day
Age 50 or older	1,200 mg per day	800–1,000 IU per day
Women who have had breast cancer	1,200 mg per day	400–600 IU per day
Sources: National Osteoporosis Foundation, American Society of Clinical Oncology		

Good Dietary Sources of Calcium and Vitamin D

Calcium
- Yogurt
  - 8 oz plain: 400 mg
  - 8 oz fruit: 250–400 mg
- Milk, 8 oz: 300 mg
- Calcium-fortified orange juice, 8 oz: 300 mg
- Canned salmon, 3 oz: 200 mg
- Cheese, 1 oz: 200 mg
- Ice cream, 8 oz: 200 mg
- Tofu, 4 oz: 200 mg
- Cottage cheese, 8 oz: 100 mg
- Cooked greens, 4 oz: 100 mg
- Cooked or dried peas or beans, 8 oz: 100 mg
- Nonfat powdered milk,1 tablespoon (add to casseroles, baked goods, puddings): 50 mg

Vitamin D
- Cooked salmon, 3.5 oz: 360 IU
- Cooked mackerel, 3.5 oz: 345 IU
- Tuna fish, canned in oil, 3 oz: 200 IU
- Ready-to-eat cereal, ¾–1 cup, fortified with 10% daily value of vitamin D: 40 IU
- Egg, 1 yolk: 20 IU

Get regular weight-bearing exercise. Exercise is weight-bearing if your feet and legs bear your body's weight while you do it. Walking, jogging, climbing stairs, dancing, and playing tennis are all examples of weight-bearing exercise. Muscle-strengthening exercises like lifting weights also help keep your bones strong.

Do not smoke. Smoking is just as bad for bones as it is for the heart and lungs.

Do not drink alcohol to excess. Heavy alcohol use may increase risk for bone loss and fractures.

Are There Treatments for Bone Loss for People With Cancer?

Medications are available that can help slow bone loss or reduce the risk of broken bones in people with osteoporosis. Some medications for bone loss, however, are best avoided if you have had cancer. They could interfere with cancer treatment or help cancer start growing again.

Talk with a member of your healthcare team about whether medication to slow bone loss is right for you. If your doctor prescribes a medication to treat bone loss, be sure to take the medication exactly as he or she tells you to.

For More Information

For additional information about bone loss and osteoporosis, see the following resources.

National Institute of Arthritis and Musculoskeletal and Skin Diseases

- What Breast Cancer Survivors Need to Know About Osteoporosis: www.niams.nih.gov/Health_Info/Bone/Osteoporosis/ Conditions_Behaviors/osteoporosis_breast_cancer.asp

- What Prostate Cancer Survivors Need to Know About Osteoporosis: www.niams.nih.gov/Health_Info/Bone/Osteoporosis/Conditions_Behaviors/osteoporosis_prostate_cancer.asp

CHAPTER 4

Breathing Difficulties

Why Do I Have a Hard Time Breathing or Get Out of Breath Very Quickly?

FEELING SHORT OF BREATH OR HAVING DIFFICULTY breathing is something that some people with cancer experience. People may describe this symptom in different ways. Some people say they feel tightness in the chest. Others say they feel as though they cannot get enough air. Even when you are resting, you may feel as though it is hard work to breathe.

The technical name for shortness of breath or difficulty breathing is *dyspnea* (DISP-nee-uh). It is a distressing symptom that can cause anxiety, which may make the shortness of breath worse. People who have lung cancer and people whose cancer has reached an advanced stage are most likely to have breathing difficulties, but breathing difficulties can occur with any cancer at any stage.

Shortness of breath may have many causes in people with cancer. Often it does not have a single cause but rather several factors that together cause it to happen. Finally, people with cancer may have other health problems, such as asthma or heart failure, prior to a cancer diagnosis that can cause shortness of breath.

Cancer itself can cause shortness of breath. A tumor or fluid buildup in the lungs or stomach may obstruct the airways, making it hard to breathe. Other cancer symptoms, such as anemia, cachexia (a condition associated with weight loss, muscle loss, fatigue, and weakness), and infection, can cause breathing difficulties. Surgery, radiation treatment, and chemotherapy can all cause shortness of breath.

Are There Tests for Shortness of Breath?

Blood tests and a test that measures the amount of oxygen in your blood can help diagnose shortness of breath. Other tests will ask you to describe or rate on a scale how hard it is for you to breathe. For example,

- On a scale of 0 to 100, how hard is it for you to breathe right now? (Zero means not at all hard, and 100 means as hard as it could be.)
- You are given a piece of paper with a line drawn on it. One end of the line is labeled "No shortness of breath." The other end is labeled "Shortness of breath as bad as it could be." Make a mark on the line at the point that best describes how bad your shortness of breath is right now.

Your doctor or nurse may ask questions to find out more about exactly when you are having breathing difficulties (see Questions You May Be Asked About Shortness of Breath).

Questions You May Be Asked About Shortness of Breath

- Are you ever troubled by shortness of breath when hurrying on level ground or walking up a slight hill?
- Do you get short of breath walking with other people at an ordinary pace on level ground?
- Do you have to stop for breath when walking at your own pace on level ground?
- Do you get short of breath when you are washing or dressing?
- Are you too short of breath to leave the house?

If you are having difficulty breathing, it is very important for you to tell a member of your healthcare team about it. If no one asks you about it, be sure to bring it up yourself.

What Treatments Are Available for Shortness of Breath?

The way shortness of breath is treated depends on what is causing it. For example, if a tumor is obstructing your airway, treatment (chemotherapy or radiation) to remove or shrink the tumor may also relieve your breathing difficulties. If you have an infection that is causing shortness of breath, treating the infection with antibiotics may help.

Opioid drugs such as morphine that are used to treat cancer pain can also be used to relieve shortness of breath. They do this by slowing down the "drive" to breathe. If anxiety is making your breathing difficulties worse, an anti-anxiety medication may help.

Some medications for shortness of breath come in a form that can be inhaled instead of swallowed as a pill. There is no evidence that inhaled medications work better than pills for most people. However, some individuals report having more relief from inhaled medications than from pills. If you are taking an inhaled medication, it is important to learn how to use the inhaler properly. A member of your healthcare team can help you do this.

Oxygen therapy helps some people feel less short of breath. Some people use oxygen therapy at night to help them breathe more easily while they sleep. Others find it helps when they are walking or doing anything that involves effort. Again, it is important to learn how to use oxygen equipment properly and safely. A member of your healthcare team can help you do this.

What Else Can I Do to Cope With Shortness of Breath Caused by Cancer or Cancer Treatment?

There are many things you can do that may help relieve shortness of breath.

- Do not smoke, and do not spend time around people who are smoking.
- Try to avoid being around anyone who has a cold or a flu-like illness.
- Try leaning forward. You can do this from either a sitting or standing position. Moving your upper body forward may help you breathe better.
- Sit near a fan or an open window. Cool air blowing across your face and into your nose may help you feel less short of breath.
- Try breathing out with pursed lips. After you inhale, position your lips as if you were going to whistle or blow out a candle, then exhale. If you find this hard to do, try holding a fist up to your mouth and exhaling through it. Do not breathe too hard as you do this. Just exhale normally.
- Try breathing through your stomach. Place one hand on your chest and the other on your stomach. Inhale slowly and feel your stomach expand with your hand. Exhale slowly. Rest, then repeat. You may find that this not only helps you breathe more easily but that it also helps you relax.
- Pace yourself. Save your energy for the most important things you need to do. Move slowly and evenly. Avoid sudden, jerky movements.
- Try relaxation therapy. For example, learn to gradually relax all the muscles in your body. Relaxation techniques may relieve stress and help take your mind off your breathing difficulties.
- Try acupuncture. In some studies, this technique helped some people with cancer get relief from shortness of breath.

For More Information

For additional information about breathing difficulties, see the following resources.

American Society of Clinical Oncology (ASCO)

- Shortness of Breath or Dyspnea—ASCO Curriculum: www. cancer.net/patient/All+About+Cancer/Treating+Cancer/ Managing+Side+Effects/Shortness+of+Breath+or+ Dyspnea+-+ASCO+curriculum

National Cancer Institute

- Dyspnea and Coughing During Advanced Cancer (PDQ®): www.cancer.gov/cancertopics/pdq/supportivecare/cardio pulmonary/Patient/page2

Oncology Nursing Society

- The Cancer Journey: Side Effects—Shortness of Breath: www .thecancerjourney.org/side/se-14

Cancer Cachexia

What Is Cancer Cachexia?

CANCER CACHEXIA (ka-KEK-see-uh) IS A WASTING condition that causes weight loss, muscle loss, fatigue, and weakness. It is common in people with cancer. Around half to three-quarters of all patients with cancer have cachexia to some extent.

What Causes Cancer Cachexia?

In some cases, cancer itself can cause cachexia. Tumors may produce chemicals that change the way the body uses the nutrients in food. Although a patient may appear to be eating enough, the body may not be able to absorb the nutrients in the food.

Cancer treatment and its side effects also may lead to cachexia. Chemotherapy and radiation may cause a loss of appetite, nausea and vomiting, mouth sores, taste changes, and other side effects. These side effects can make it hard to eat enough food to meet your body's needs.

Also, if you are having pain or feeling tired all the time because of your cancer treatment, you may be less active than you used to be. Lack of activity can lead to muscle wasting and loss of strength.

What Are the Symptoms of Cancer Cachexia?

Loss of appetite, or anorexia, is usually the most noticeable symptom. You may also find that food just does not taste as good as it used to, or that you feel full after eating very little. Patients experiencing cachexia will also have weight loss (see Symptoms of Cancer Cachexia).

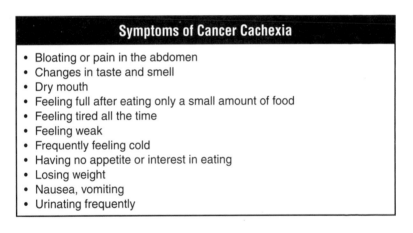

Symptoms of Cancer Cachexia

- Bloating or pain in the abdomen
- Changes in taste and smell
- Dry mouth
- Feeling full after eating only a small amount of food
- Feeling tired all the time
- Feeling weak
- Frequently feeling cold
- Having no appetite or interest in eating
- Losing weight
- Nausea, vomiting
- Urinating frequently

Can Cancer Cachexia Be Prevented?

It is hard to prevent cancer cachexia entirely, but you may be able to stop it from becoming serious. These tips may help you halt more weight and muscle loss and maintain your current level of activity.

- Eat frequent, small meals.
- Eat foods high in protein and calories (for example, whole milk, ice cream, pudding, cheese, peanut butter, fruit juice, dried fruit).

- Eat as much as you can at breakfast.
- Eat meals with family and friends.
- See a dietitian for help preparing an eating plan that meets your needs.
- Get regular exercise. It will strengthen your muscles and help you feel better. Increasing your activity level may help stimulate your appetite.

How Is Cancer Cachexia Treated?

Your doctor may prescribe a medication to increase your appetite. If you find it hard to chew or swallow, your doctor may suggest that you be fed through a tube placed in your stomach or intestine.

There is a lack of evidence to support the use of dietary supplements such as omega-3 fatty acids, growth hormone and other steroids, and melatonin in treating cancer cachexia.

Hydrazine sulfate, another dietary supplement, is not recommended for cancer cachexia. Cancer researchers have done several studies in which some patients took hydrazine sulfate and others took a placebo or "sugar pill." In most of these studies, the patients who took hydrazine sulfate did not have any better appetite or gain any more weight than those who took the placebo.

The drug Marinol® (dronabinol) is a marijuana derivative that is approved in the United States to treat appetite and weight loss in patients with AIDS. Studies with Marinol in patients with cancer have so far had mixed results. In some studies, patients with cancer taking Marinol had a better appetite and gain weight. In other studies, however, Marinol had no effect on patients' appetite or weight.

For More Information

For additional information about cancer cachexia, see the following resources.

American Cancer Society

• Nutrition for People With Cancer: www.cancer.org/Treatment/SurvivorshipDuringandAfterTreatment/NutritionforPeoplewithCancer/index

American Society of Clinical Oncology

• Appetite Loss: www.cancer.net/patient/Coping/Emotional+and+Physical+Matters/Managing+Side+Effects/Appetite+Loss

National Cancer Institute

• Nutrition in Cancer Care (PDQ®): www.cancer.gov/cancertopics/pdq/supportivecare/nutrition/Patient/page1

Oncology Nursing Society

• The Cancer Journey: Side Effects—Appetite/Weight Loss (Anorexia): www.thecancerjourney.org/side/se-2

Cancer Pain

What Causes Cancer Pain?

MANY PEOPLE WITH CANCER HAVE PAIN. THE cancer itself can cause pain, especially if it grows and spreads to the bones or other organs. Cancer treatment can also cause pain.

It is common to have pain after cancer surgery. This type of pain usually goes away as your body heals. Radiation and chemotherapy often cause pain, too. This type of pain may go away once treatment is finished. In some cases, however, treatment may cause nerve damage that does not heal. The area with the nerve damage may remain painful long after treatment is over. Some people who have had radiation to the chest, breast, or spinal cord can develop pain at the treatment site months or years later.

Some cancer pain is *persistent* or *chronic* (it never goes away or lasts a long time). Some cancer pain comes and goes. It may flare up suddenly even if you are taking pain medication. This is called *breakthrough pain* because it "breaks through" your pain treatment.

Do I Just Have to Put Up With Cancer Pain?

People sometimes think they have no choice but to be tolerant of cancer pain—this is absolutely false. Having cancer is stressful enough without pain. Untreated pain can make you feel miserable. It can also keep you from sleeping well and from being active. It is hard to think clearly and make decisions when you are in pain. Untreated pain makes life harder not only for you but also for those who care for you and about you.

The good news is that cancer pain can almost always be relieved. If you are having pain from your cancer or its treatment, talk with a member of your healthcare team about it. Every time you visit your doctor's office, someone should ask you if you are having any pain (see Questions You May Be Asked About Cancer Pain). If you are having pain but no one asks you about it, do not leave the office without talking to someone about it.

Questions You May Be Asked About Cancer Pain

Questions About Persistent Pain
- When did the pain start?
- What does the pain feel like? What words would you use to describe your pain?
- Where is your pain? Show me where it hurts.
- On a scale of 0 to 10—with 0 being no pain and 10 being the worst pain you can imagine—how much does it hurt right now? How much does it hurt when the pain is at its worst?
- Using this scale (none, mild, moderate, severe, intolerable), tell me how much your pain hurts right now and how much it hurts at its worst.
- What makes your pain better? What makes it worse?
- What treatments have you tried to relieve your pain? How well have they worked?
- How does your pain affect
  - Your mood?
  - Your ability to do your usual daily activities?
  - Your sleep?
  - Your ability to spend time with family members and friends?
  - Your sex life?

Questions About Breakthrough Pain
- Do you have sudden flare-ups of pain that come and go, "breaking through" your pain treatment?

(Continued on next page)

(Continued)

Questions You May Be Asked About Cancer Pain

- How many sudden flare-ups of pain do you have in a day? How long do these flare-ups last?
- Are you having a flare-up of pain right now? On a scale of 0 to 10— with 0 being no pain and 10 being the worst pain you can imagine— how much does it hurt right now? How much does it hurt when the pain is at its worst?
- Using this scale (none, mild, moderate, severe, intolerable), tell me how much your pain hurts right now and how much it hurts at its worst.
- Do you have flare-ups of pain when you move or when you are active? Do you have flare-ups of pain that "just happen"?
- What treatments have you tried to relieve pain flare-ups? How well have the treatments worked?
- How do pain flare-ups affect
  - Your mood?
  - Your ability to do your usual daily activities?
  - Your sleep?
  - Your ability to spend time with family members and friends?
  - Your sex life?

How Is Cancer Pain Treated?

Several different kinds of medication can be used to treat cancer pain. It may take some time to find the pain medication that works best for you. Often, taking two kinds of pain medication works better than taking just one kind (see Examples of Medications That May Be Used to Treat Cancer Pain).

Examples of Medications That May Be Used to Treat Cancer Pain

Type	Examples	Description
Anticonvulsants	• Gabapentin (Neurontin®) • Pregabalin (Lyrica®)	These medications are used to treat seizures as well as to relieve pain caused by nerve damage.

(Continued on next page)

(Continued)

Examples of Medications That May Be Used to Treat Cancer Pain

Type	Examples	Description

Analgesics	• Acetaminophen (Anacin®, Tylenol®)
	• Nonsteroidal anti-inflammatory drugs, including
	  – Aspirin (Bayer®, Bufferin®, Excedrin®)
	  – Celecoxib (Celebrex®)
	  – Ibuprofen (Advil®, Motrin®)
	  – Indomethacin (Indocin®)
	  – Naproxen (Aleve®, Naprosyn®)
	  – Sulindac (Clinoril®)
	• Opioids, including
	  – Fentanyl (Duragesic®)
	  – Hydrocodone (Vicodin®)
	  – Hydromorphone (Dilaudid®)
	  – Morphine sulfate (MS Contin® CR [continuous release])
	  – Oxycodone (OxyContin®)
		The primary use of these medications is to relieve pain.

Corticosteroids	• Dexamethasone (Decadron®) • Prednisone	These medications may be used to treat pain as well as for many other purposes, including treating cancer.
Tricyclic antidepressants	• Desipramine (Norpramin®) • Doxepin (Sinequan®) • Imipramine (Tofranil®) • Nortriptyline (Aventyl®, Pamelor®)	The primary use of these medications is to treat depression, but they may also be used for pain relief.

I Am Afraid of Becoming Addicted to Pain Medication.

You are not alone; many people with cancer worry about becoming addicted to medications in the class of drugs known as opioids (OH-pee-oyds). These medications are very effective at relieving chronic or persistent cancer pain. Concerns about addiction may arise because of confusion about three concepts: addiction, physical dependence, and tolerance.

People who are addicted to a drug are unable to control their use of it. They crave the drug and continue to use it even when drug use harms their bodies, keeps them from holding a job, and causes serious problems in their personal lives. It is extremely rare for people who use opioids for pain relief to become addicted to them.

Physical dependence on a drug is not the same as addiction. Many kinds of medication, including pain medications, cause changes in your body when you take them. If you stop taking the medication suddenly, you will feel unpleasant withdrawal symptoms. This is *not* a sign of addiction. It means your body has become used to the presence of the drug and is reacting to its sudden withdrawal.

You can avoid withdrawal symptoms by slowly reducing the dose of a medication so your body has time to reverse the changes the drug caused. Work closely with your doctor when reducing the dose of any medication.

Tolerance means that over time you may need to take a higher dose of a medication to get the same effect. This is normal and is *not* a sign of addiction. In fact, many people do not develop tolerance to the pain-relieving effects of opioid medications. Once they are on an effective dose, they can usually stay on the same dose for a long time.

The key to avoiding addiction is to take your medication exactly as your doctor prescribes. Most people who take their pain medication as directed by their doctor do not become addicted. If you are worried about becoming addicted to your pain medication, share your concerns with a member of your healthcare team.

What Side Effects Can Opioid Medications Cause?

Constipation is the most common side effect of opioid medications. When your doctor prescribes an opioid for you, he or she should also start you on treatment to prevent constipation. (See Chapter 9 for more about treating constipation in people with cancer.)

You may feel sleepy for the first few days after you start taking an opioid. You may also throw up or feel like you are going to throw up. Your doctor may prescribe other medications to treat these side effects. These side effects usually wear off once you are on a stable dose of an opioid medication. Then you can stop taking the other medications.

What Else Can I Do to Cope With Cancer Pain?

Relaxation and breathing exercises can help you feel less tense and anxious about cancer pain. Massaging the area where you have pain, or applying hot or cold packs to it, also may help. In addition, you may want to try listening to relaxing music or using guided imagery to take your mind off the pain.

For More Information

For additional information about cancer pain, see the following resources.

American Cancer Society

- Cancer Pain: Don't Suffer in Silence: www.cancer.org/Cancer/news/Features/cancer-pain-dont-suffer-in-silence

American Society of Clinical Oncology (ASCO)

- Pain—ASCO Curriculum: www.cancer.net/patient/All+About
  +Cancer/Treating+Cancer/Managing+Side+Effects/Pain+
  -+ASCO+curriculum

National Cancer Institute

- Pain Control: Support for People With Cancer: www.cancer
  .gov/cancertopics/paincontrol/page1

Oncology Nursing Society

- The Cancer Journey: Side Effects—Pain: www.thecancer
  journey.org/side/se-13

CHAPTER 7

Cancer-Related Fatigue

What Is Cancer-Related Fatigue?

FATIGUE MEANS FEELING TIRED. CANCER-RELATED fatigue, however, is not the same as the tiredness you normally feel after a long day. You may feel tired, weak, and low on energy all the time. Even after a night's sleep, you may still feel deeply tired. Any activity, such as walking around the house or making a simple meal, may leave you feeling exhausted. You may feel so tired that you cannot work, take part in family activities, or do any of the things you usually do.

Fatigue is one of the most common symptoms in people with cancer. Although it is very common, it affects everyone differently. People may describe their feelings of fatigue in different ways. For example, some people may say they feel tired, weary, or weak, or that their arms and legs feel heavy. Others may complain that they feel mentally "foggy," want to sleep all the time, or do not sleep well.

Many people find that their fatigue goes away once they have completed their cancer treatment. Others, however, may continue to feel weak and tired for a long time after their treatment is over.

Although fatigue is a common and distressing symptom for people with cancer, it is not a symptom that patients or their healthcare providers talk about as much. Patients may think it is just something they have to put up with, so they do not mention it when talking to their healthcare team. But ways to effectively treat cancer-related fatigue are available. If you are suffering from cancer-related fatigue, be sure to talk with your healthcare team about it and ask what can be done to relieve your fatigue.

What Causes Fatigue in People With Cancer?

In most cases, cancer-related fatigue has no single cause. Both cancer and cancer treatment disrupt the body's normal functioning in a variety of ways that can trigger fatigue. For example, chemotherapy and radiation therapy can cause the body to produce toxic substances that alter how cells in the body work. Some of these changes may result in feelings of extreme fatigue.

Cancer or its treatment may interfere with the body's ability to make red blood cells, causing anemia (see Chapter 1). A persistent feeling of tiredness and low energy is the most common symptom of anemia.

You may also feel sleepy or tired as a side effect of using certain medications (see Examples of Medications That May Cause Sleepiness or Fatigue).

Examples of Medications That May Cause Sleepiness or Fatigue
• Anti-allergy medications
• Anti-anxiety medications
– Buspirone (Buspar®)
– Lorazepam (Ativan®)
• Antidepressants
• Antiemetics (medications that prevent or relieve nausea and vomiting)

(Continued on next page)

(Continued)

Examples of Medications That May Cause Sleepiness or Fatigue

• Antiseizure medications
  – Carbamazepine (Tegretol®)
  – Gabapentin (Neurontin®)
  – Phenobarbital
• Medications that slow the heart rate
• Opioid pain medications
  – Morphine
  – Oxycodone
  – Hydromorphone
• Sedatives (drugs that relieve anxiety or help with sleep)

It is normal to feel extremely tired during the first few days of a chemotherapy treatment cycle. After that, feelings of fatigue often slowly improve until the next treatment cycle begins. With radiation treatment, fatigue may get worse as treatment continues and the worst fatigue may be felt at the end of or after treatment is over.

Patients who have fatigue may have other symptoms as well, such as breathing difficulties, disturbed sleep, loss of appetite, and pain.

How Do I Know if I Have Cancer-Related Fatigue?

There are no blood tests or other laboratory tests to diagnose cancer-related fatigue. How you feel is the most important factor in diagnosing cancer-related fatigue. While you are going through treatment for your cancer, a member of your healthcare team should ask you questions from time to time about how tired you are feeling (see Questions That Help to Identify Cancer-Related Fatigue).

If you are feeling much more tired than usual during your cancer treatment, but no one from your healthcare team asks you about it, be sure to bring the subject up yourself.

Questions That Help to Identify Cancer-Related Fatigue

- On a scale of 0 to 10—where 0 is not tired at all and 10 is the worst tiredness you can imagine—how bad would you say your fatigue has been during the past week?
- Would you say that your fatigue is mild, moderate, or severe?
- When did you start feeling tired?
- How often do you feel tired? (How many hours per day or days per week?)
- How much have you limited social activities, found it hard to get things done, or found it hard to keep a positive outlook because of feeling tired?
- How does feeling tired affect your relationships, your ability to work, and your ability to do things at home?
- What makes your fatigue better?
- What makes your fatigue worse?
- What do you do to cope with fatigue?
- Does rest relieve your fatigue?
- Do you have trouble sleeping?
- Do you have other symptoms (difficulty breathing, pain, nausea, vomiting)?
- Do you ever feel anxious? If yes, how often?
- Do you feel discouraged, blue, or sad? If yes, how often?
- Have you talked about your fatigue with anyone on your healthcare team?
- Has anyone given you any tips for coping with fatigue?

What Can Be Done to Treat Fatigue in People With Cancer?

The most effective treatments for fatigue in people with cancer are coping strategies and lifestyle changes. As yet, no medications have been found to be consistently helpful for most people with cancer-related fatigue.

Understanding that cancer or its treatment often causes fatigue may help you cope better with this symptom. Fatigue does not necessarily mean your cancer treatment is not working or your cancer is getting worse.

Try recording in a diary when you feel tired and what makes your fatigue better or worse. This may help you better understand how fatigue affects you. Talking with a member of your healthcare team or with other people with cancer in a support group may help you feel more able to cope with fatigue.

Studies show that regular exercise is a very good way to relieve fatigue. Talk with a member of your healthcare team about how much and what kind of exercise you can safely do. Start slowly. At first, a few minutes of activity a day may be all you can do. As you become stronger, you will be able to do more each day.

These strategies may also help you cope with cancer-related fatigue:

- Find ways to conserve energy as you go about your daily routines (see How to Cope With Fatigue by Conserving Energy).
- Adopt healthy sleep habits (see Healthy Sleep Habits).
- Eat a healthy, balanced diet and drink plenty of fluids.
- Try yoga, massage, music therapy, and other alternative therapies to help you relax.

How to Cope With Fatigue by Conserving Energy

Try these tips to see which ones you find helpful.
- Rearrange your environment.
  - Keep items you use often in places where you can reach them easily.
  - Adjust work spaces (for example, raise a table top) so that you are not sitting or standing awkwardly. Bad posture wastes energy.
  - Sit rather than stand whenever possible (for example, while preparing meals or washing dishes).

(Continued on next page)

(Continued)

How to Cope With Fatigue by Conserving Energy

- – Use tools and assistive devices to make tasks easier. For example, use a jar opener to get tight-fitting lids off containers. Instead of standing on a chair to get something down from a high shelf, use a reaching tool. Get a shower chair so that you can sit in the tub or shower.
  - – Soak dishes before washing them. Then let the dishes air dry. Or use paper plates and napkins.
  - – Use prepared foods instead of making meals from scratch.
  - – Use a rolling cart to carry things around the house.
  - – Ask if your grocery store will deliver your groceries.
  - – When you shop, ask the store for a wheelchair or scooter.
- Plan ahead.
  - – Before starting a task or project, gather all the supplies you will need in one place.
  - – Call ahead to stores to find out if the items you want are in stock.
  - – When you cook, make more than you need for one meal. Freeze the extra portions for later.
  - – Take rest breaks during activities. Take a break *before* you feel tired.
  - – Allow enough time to complete a task without rushing. Rushing uses more energy.
  - – Keep a daily journal for a few weeks to identify tasks that are tiring or times of day when you are more likely to feel tired.
- Set priorities.
  - – Identify tasks that are less important to you. Then just do not do them, or do them less often.
  - – Give tasks to family members or friends who offer to help.
  - – Consider hiring help (for example, a cleaning service, a lawn service) to reduce your workload.
- Alternate activity with rest.
  - – Avoid bursts of activity or long periods of activity that tire you out.
  - – With your healthcare team's okay, start a program of regular exercise (for example, walking or cycling). Begin by doing 5 or 10 minutes of activity twice a day if you can. Increase the time by one minute every day.
  - – Try to exercise regularly and consistently, but do not overdo it.
- Avoid long naps during the day.
- Do not nap in the late afternoon.
- Go to bed only when you feel sleepy.

Healthy Sleep Habits
• Do not read or work on a laptop computer in bed. • Do not lie in bed awake. If you cannot fall asleep, get out of bed until you feel sleepy. • Go to bed and get up at about the same time every day. • Avoid caffeinated beverages in the evening. • Relax for an hour before going to bed. • Adopt a routine that you use every night before going to bed.

For More Information

For additional information about cancer-related fatigue, see the following resources.

American Cancer Society

• Fatigue in People With Cancer: www.cancer.org/Treatment/ TreatmentsandSideEffects/PhysicalSideEffects/Fatigue/ FatigueinPeoplewithCancer/index?sitearea=MIT

American Society of Clinical Oncology (ASCO)

• Fatigue—ASCO Curriculum: www.cancer.net/patient/All +About+Cancer/Treating+Cancer/Managing+Side+Effects/ Fatigue+-+ASCO+curriculum

Oncology Nursing Society

• The Cancer Journey: Side Effects—Fatigue: www.thecancer journey.org/side/se-8

Changes in Sexuality

How Can Cancer Affect My Sex Life?

CANCER OR ITS TREATMENT CAN AFFECT YOUR sex life in several ways. Some of these changes are temporary. In other cases, the changes can be long-lasting.

- Women may be unable to become pregnant.
- Men may be unable to father children.
- Men may not be able to have an erection.
- Women may have less vaginal secretion or lubrication.
- Having sex may be painful.
- Both men and women may lose the desire to have sex.
- Both men and women may feel less sexually attractive because they have had cancer.

Why Does Cancer or Its Treatment Cause Changes in Sexuality?

Surgery, radiation, and chemotherapy can all affect the body in ways that can interfere with having sex. For example, surgery for prostate cancer may damage nerves and muscles that affect the penis. This damage can prevent a man from having an erection. Trouble getting an erection is called erectile dysfunction (ED).

Most men who have surgery to remove the prostate gland will have ED afterward. It may take 18 months to 2 years after prostate cancer surgery for ED to go away.

Radiation treatment for prostate cancer can also cause ED. In this case, the problem usually comes on slowly during the first year after treatment.

The effects of cancer and its treatment on the ability to have children are a special concern for young people with cancer. In both men and women, cancer treatment may damage the reproductive organs.

For example, many drugs used to treat breast cancer stop a woman's monthly periods. Depending on the woman's age and other factors, her periods may or may not return to normal after cancer treatment is over. Radiation therapy also can damage a woman's reproductive organs. Both surgery and radiation can damage a man's sperm so that he cannot father a child.

Surgery, chemotherapy, and hormonal therapy can cause a loss of desire for sex. People with cancer also may lose the desire for sex because of other symptoms like fatigue (see Chapter 7), depression (see Chapter 10), and nausea or vomiting (see Chapter 18). Damage to the reproductive organs may cause changes that make having sex painful for both men and women.

Cancer and its treatment may cause physical changes such as the loss of a body part, a change in the shape of a body part, a loss or gain in weight, or hair loss (see Chapter 12). People with cancer may feel less sexually attractive because of these changes.

Also, having cancer and being treated for cancer can cause anxiety and stress, not only for you but also for your partner. This can put a strain on many aspects of your life, including your sex life.

Why Should I Talk About My Sex Life With My Doctor When I'm Embarrassed? Is It Really *That* Important?

Many people feel awkward discussing sex with their healthcare providers. It is also common to feel you should not complain about a "minor" problem such as a change in your sex life when it is a side effect of life-saving cancer treatment. However, not talking about it does not make the problem go away.

A healthy sex life is an important part of a healthy life for many people. Feeling unhappy or anxious about a change in your sex life is nothing to be ashamed of. If a change in your sex life is bothering you, do not suffer in silence and shame. Talk to a member of your healthcare team about it.

What Can Be Done About Changes in Sexuality Caused by Cancer or Cancer Treatment?

An important first step is to understand that changes in sexuality are common in people with cancer. These changes affect both you and your partner. Both of you should talk with your healthcare team about what sexual side effects your treatment may cause, how long they might last, and how they can be treated. Treatment options will vary depending on the type of problem.

Sharing your concerns can be helpful. In addition to talking with a member of your healthcare team, consider joining a support group or getting counseling. In addition, treating other cancer symptoms like depression or fatigue may improve sexual side effects.

Your sex life may change after cancer diagnosis and treatment, but sex can continue to be an enjoyable part of your life. Reassure your partner that cancer has not changed how you feel about him or her. Try exploring new ways to be intimate with each other.

Women may find that Kegel exercises, which strengthen the muscles below the pelvis, are helpful to ease a lack of sexual desire or pain during sex. Your healthcare provider can explain how to do these exercises. Products that lubricate the vagina may also help; however, women who have had breast cancer should not use lubricants that contain estrogen. Water-soluble lubricants are preferred. Women may participate in programs such as the "Look Good ... Feel Better®" program, which shows women how to wear wigs and makeup to help with feeling more attractive.

Some changes in sexuality can be treated with medication. Be sure to take the medication exactly as your doctor tells you to. Avoid buying pills for sexual problems over the Internet. Also, do not cut pills in half or take pills that someone else gives you.

For young people with cancer, it is important before treatment starts to explore options for preserving the ability to have children in the future. This is known as *fertility preservation*. Options may include freezing sperm, eggs, or embryos. Procedures that protect the reproductive organs from radiation also may help. Talk with your healthcare team about what options for fertility preservation may be right for you.

For More Information

For additional information about changes in sexuality, see the following resources.

American Cancer Society

- Sex and Men With Cancer: www.cancer.org/Treatment/ TreatmentsandSideEffects/PhysicalSideEffects/Sexual SideEffectsinMen/SexandMenwithCancer/index

- Sex and Women With Cancer: www.cancer.org/Treatment/ TreatmentsandSideEffects/PhysicalSideEffects/Sexual SideEffectsinWomen/SexandWomenwithCancer/index

Hygeia Media, an imprint of the Oncology Nursing Society

- *Man Cancer Sex,* by Anne Katz: http://esource.ons.org/ ProductDetails.aspx?sku=INPU0603
- *Woman Cancer Sex,* by Anne Katz: http://esource.ons.org/ productDetails.aspx?sku=INPU0595

Look Good … Feel Better®

- Free, nonmedical, brand-neutral, national public service program to help people with cancer manage their treatment and recovery: www.lookgoodfeelbetter.org

National Cancer Institute

- What Men Can Do About Changes in Sexuality and Fertility: www.cancer.gov/cancertopics/wtk/men-fertility
- What Women Can Do About Changes in Sexuality and Fertility: www.cancer.gov/cancertopics/wtk/women-fertility

Constipation

What Is Constipation?

CONSTIPATION MEANS HAVING BOWEL MOVE-ments that are less frequent than is usual for you and are hard to pass. You may have pain when you pass the stool. You may also feel bloating or cramping in your stomach.

People often think they are constipated if they do not have a bowel movement every day. Although some people have a bowel movement daily, others have bowel movements less frequently. Everyone is different. As a general rule, you should have at least three bowel movements a week.

What Causes Constipation in People With Cancer?

Constipation can have a number of causes in people with cancer. Cancer itself can cause constipation if, for example, a tumor is blocking the bowel. Some chemotherapy drugs can cause constipation. Many other kinds of medication (including drugs often used to relieve pain in people with cancer) can also cause constipation (see Medications That Can Cause Constipation).

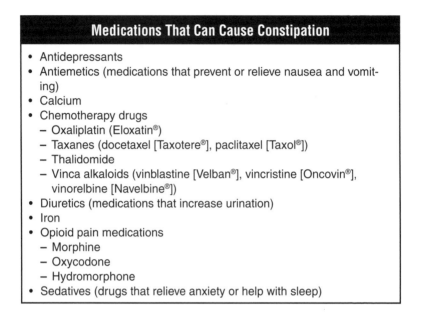

Medications That Can Cause Constipation

- Antidepressants
- Antiemetics (medications that prevent or relieve nausea and vomiting)
- Calcium
- Chemotherapy drugs
  - Oxaliplatin (Eloxatin®)
  - Taxanes (docetaxel [Taxotere®], paclitaxel [Taxol®])
  - Thalidomide
  - Vinca alkaloids (vinblastine [Velban®], vincristine [Oncovin®], vinorelbine [Navelbine®])
- Diuretics (medications that increase urination)
- Iron
- Opioid pain medications
  - Morphine
  - Oxycodone
  - Hydromorphone
- Sedatives (drugs that relieve anxiety or help with sleep)

People with cancer can become constipated if they are eating poorly or drinking too little liquid. Reduced physical activity and even sadness or anxiety about cancer or its treatment can also lead to constipation. Another possible cause is scarring of the bowel as a result of surgery or radiation treatment.

Can Constipation During Cancer Treatment Be Prevented?

The best way to deal with constipation during cancer treatment is to prevent it from developing in the first place. Talk with a member of your healthcare team about steps you can take to reduce your risk of constipation (see Diet and Lifestyle Steps That Can Reduce the Risk of Constipation).

Diet and Lifestyle Steps That Can Reduce the Risk of Constipation

- If you can, eat foods that are high in fiber (fruits, vegetables, bran, whole-grain breads and cereals). Fiber makes stools bulkier and softer so they are easier to pass. If you are not used to eating high-fiber foods, add them to your diet gradually to avoid bloating and gas. (If you have had a bowel obstruction or bowel surgery, you should not eat foods high in fiber.)
- Drink at least eight 8-oz. servings of liquid every day. Some of these servings should be warm or hot liquids (coffee, tea, warm water), which help stimulate the bowel.
- Be as physically active as you are able to be. Walking is an excellent way to stay active. Talk with a member of your healthcare team about setting up an exercise program that is right for you. Being active also helps stimulate the bowel.
- Try to plan to have a bowel movement after you have eaten a meal. The muscles in your gut are most active after you eat, so that is when you are most likely to get the urge to have a bowel movement. Be careful with trying to "force" a bowel movement when constipated, as this can lead to hemorrhoids.
- When you feel the urge to have a bowel movement, do not ignore it or suppress it. Get to a bathroom as quickly as you can.

How Are People With Cancer Treated for Constipation?

Sometimes lifestyle steps are not enough to prevent constipation. In that case, or if you are taking medications that cause constipation, treatment with laxatives and stool softeners is the next step. Laxatives are drugs that stimulate the bowels to move. (If you have an obstructed bowel, however, you should not take laxatives.) Stool softeners make the stool less firm and easier to pass. Of special importance, people taking opioid narcotics for pain should also be on a bowel regimen of laxatives.

Several kinds of laxatives are available, and they work in different ways. Treatment with two different laxatives is often more effective than treatment with just one. Talk with a member of your healthcare team about the laxative regimen that is right for you.

Take laxatives as directed by your doctor. Do not take more of them than your doctor tells you to. It is also important to stop taking laxatives if the stool turns to diarrhea or becomes too loose.

If you become severely constipated, you may need to have an enema to remove the stool and cleanse the colon. Taking a medication for pain or anxiety before this procedure may help to make it less uncomfortable.

For More Information

For additional information about constipation, see the following resources.

American Cancer Society

- Constipation: www.cancer.org/Treatment/TreatmentsandSide Effects/PhysicalSideEffects/DealingwithSymptomsatHome/ caring-for-the-patient-with-cancer-at-home-constipation

National Cancer Institute

- Gastrointestinal Complications (PDQ®): Constipation: www .cancer.gov/cancertopics/pdq/supportivecare/gastrointestinal complications/Patient/page3

Oncology Nursing Society

- The Cancer Journey: Side Effects—Constipation: www. thecancerjourney.org/side/se-5

10

Depression

What Is Depression?

D EPRESSION IS AN INTENSE LOW MOOD OR FEEL-
ing of despair that lasts for at least two weeks. A person
who is depressed loses interest in most of the activities
he or she used to enjoy.

Depression is common in some people with cancer. As many
as one out of four people with cancer may also have depression.

It is normal, of course, to feel sad, anxious, afraid, or de-
spairing when you learn you have cancer. With time, however, many people are able to adjust to the changes in their lives
brought on by a cancer diagnosis. Nothing will ever be exactly the same again, of course. But, gradually, many people find
they can go on with their everyday lives while they undergo
cancer treatment.

Depression is not a normal response to a cancer diagnosis. It
is a feeling of despair or hopelessness that does not go away. People who are depressed often do not have the energy to do any of
the things they normally do. They may be unable to make decisions. They may be preoccupied with thoughts of death.

Depression is an illness. It is not something you can "snap
out of." Most importantly, it is not a personal failing. Doctors
use the terms *major depression* or *clinical depression* to distinguish

the illness of depression from normal feelings of sadness or a blue mood (see Symptoms of Major Depression).

Symptoms of Major Depression

• Despairing mood
• Loss of interest in most activities that used to be enjoyable
• Persistence for at least two weeks of four or more of the following:
   – Change in appetite or weight (eating a lot more or less than usual, gaining or losing weight)
   – Change in sleep (sleeping a lot more or less than usual, waking frequently)
   – Unable to focus on a task
   – Unable to make decisions
   – Feeling tired
   – Feeling agitated
   – Thinking often about death or suicide

What Causes Depression?

Most doctors now think that depression is an illness caused by an imbalance of chemicals, known as neurotransmitters, in the brain. A risk for depression can run in families. People can become depressed, however, without having a family history of depression. Many medications (including some chemotherapy drugs) can also cause depression (see Some Examples of Medications That Can Cause Depression).

Some Examples of Medications That Can Cause Depression

• Anti-arrhythmics (medications to treat irregular heart rhythm)
• Antihistamines (medications to treat hay fever and other allergies)
• Antihypertensives (medications to treat high blood pressure)
• Chemotherapy drugs
   – Interferon
   – Steroids (for example, dexamethasone, prednisone)

(Continued on next page)

(Continued)

Some Examples of Medications That Can Cause Depression

– Tamoxifen (Nolvadex®)
  – Thalidomide (Thalomid®)
  – Vinca alkaloids (vinblastine, vincristine, vinorelbine)
• Nonsteroidal anti-inflammatory drugs
  – Celecoxib (Celebrex®)
  – Ibuprofen (Advil®, Motrin®)
  – Sulindac (Clinoril®)

How Are People With Cancer Treated for Depression?

Depression can be treated with medication and with "talk therapy" or counseling. Many different antidepressant medications are available. Some of them work by altering the balance of chemicals in the brain.

If you do not like the idea of taking antidepressants, try thinking about it this way: Taking medication for depression is just like taking insulin for diabetes. When you have diabetes, your body cannot make or use insulin properly. People with diabetes often need to take insulin every day to correct this problem.

In the same way, when you have depression, your brain does not have the right mix of chemicals it needs to function normally. Just as there is nothing to be ashamed of in taking insulin for diabetes, there is nothing to be ashamed of in taking an antidepressant for depression.

Counseling can help people with depression recognize and change patterns of negative thinking that are causing them distress. For many people with depression, a combination of medication and counseling is most helpful.

Understanding your cancer, the plan for treating it, and how to manage your symptoms may help you feel less depressed and more "in control." It may also help to remind yourself that being depressed does *not* mean there is something wrong with you as a person. Depression is an illness that can be treated.

Some people try to relieve depression by taking herbal remedies and dietary supplements. There is no evidence that these remedies are helpful for depression, and some of them, such as the herb St. John's wort, may prevent chemotherapy drugs or other medications from working properly. Tell a member of your healthcare team if you are taking any over-the-counter products such as vitamins, herbs, or other supplements, as they may block the action of your treatment.

Activities that help you relax (exercise, yoga, meditation, guided imagery, listening to calming music) may help you feel less depressed. To date, studies have not shown that any of these approaches are effective for most people with depression.

I Am Not Sure It Is Worth Going on With My Cancer Treatment. What Should I Do?

Talk with a member of your healthcare team right away if you are not sleeping well, have no energy, or have lost your appetite. When you have cancer, it is normal to sometimes feel distressed. If these feelings persist and you start to feel there is no point in going on, you may be suffering from depression. Symptoms such as poor sleep and loss of appetite can have other causes when you have cancer. It is important to tell a member of your healthcare team how you are feeling so your healthcare team can determine the cause and treat these symptoms.

One of the best things you can do for yourself when you are feeling depressed is to talk about it. Studies show that talking about your concerns can help to relieve them. Many people who are facing cancer find it helpful to meet and talk with others facing the same diagnosis. Talk with a member of your healthcare team about joining a support group.

Finally, if you feel like you might physically hurt yourself or commit suicide, it is important that you talk with your healthcare team or family members immediately.

For More Information

For additional information about depression, see the following resources.

American Cancer Society

• Anxiety, Fear, and Depression: www.cancer.org/Treatment/ TreatmentsandSideEffects/EmotionalSideEffects/Anxiety FearandDepression/index?sitearea=MBC

American Society of Clinical Oncology

• Depression and Anxiety: www.cancer.net/patient/Coping/ Emotional+and+Physical+Matters/Depression+and+Anxiety ?sectionTitle=Depression&sectionId=104465&vgnext refresh=1

National Cancer Institute

• Depression (PDQ®): www.cancer.gov/cancertopics/pdq/ supportivecare/depression/Patient/page1

Oncology Nursing Society

• Side Effects: Depression: www.thecancerjourney.org/side/ se-6

Diarrhea

What Is Diarrhea?

D IARRHEA MEANS PASSING VERY SOFT, WATERY stool more than three times in a day. The stool may or may not be bloody. You may feel a need to pass stool very urgently. You may have pain or cramps in your stomach, as well as pain or tenderness in your rectum.

Diarrhea is a very common symptom in people with cancer. People who are receiving treatment with chemotherapy or radiation are likely to get diarrhea at some point.

What Causes Diarrhea in People With Cancer?

Your intestines usually absorb most of the liquid that reaches them from your digestive system. This liquid contains nutrients and minerals such as salt and calcium that your heart, kidneys, and other organs need to function properly.

When you have cancer, or are having cancer treatment, your intestines may become damaged and may not be able to absorb liquid normally. When this happens, you will pass stool that still has a lot of liquid in it.

Some types of cancer can cause diarrhea. Surgery and radiation treatment can also cause diarrhea, as can many chemotherapy drugs and other medications used in cancer treatment. When you are being treated for cancer, you may have a higher risk for infections that can cause diarrhea. Diarrhea may also be a side effect of the drugs used to treat an infection.

Some herbal remedies and dietary supplements can cause diarrhea. Always tell a member of your healthcare team if you are taking any over-the-counter products like vitamins, herbs, or other supplements.

Doesn't Diarrhea Usually Go Away After a Couple of Days? Do I Need to Tell Anyone About It?

Always tell a member of your healthcare team right away if you have diarrhea. Diarrhea that is not treated can have severe effects on people with cancer, such as dehydration (see Serious Side Effects of Diarrhea in People With Cancer).

Serious Side Effects of Diarrhea in People With Cancer
It is a good idea to tell a member of your healthcare team as soon as you have any diarrhea. If you have any of these symptoms along with diarrhea, contact a member of your healthcare team immediately: • Bloody stools • Dizziness • Extreme thirst • Fever • Pain in the rectum • Rapid or irregular heart beat • Severe stomach cramps

When your body loses a lot of water because of diarrhea, you can quickly become dehydrated. Your heart, kidneys, and other organs may start to not work well because of the loss of minerals with the body water.

Also, when you have diarrhea, your body will not absorb your medications properly. This can quickly lead to symptoms of a medication overdose.

Call a member of your healthcare team if diarrhea does not stop after you begin taking anti-diarrheal medication.

Can I Do Anything to Prevent Diarrhea?

It is not always possible to prevent diarrhea, but you can take steps to keep it from becoming serious (see Eating and Drinking Dos and Don'ts to Help Prevent Diarrhea.).

Eating and Drinking Dos and Don'ts to Help Prevent Diarrhea

Do
- Drink 8–10 large glasses of clear liquids every day. For example, drink weak tea or clear broth (not too hot), gelatin, drinks containing glucose, or sports drinks.
- Drink liquids that replace lost nutrients and minerals (for example, Pedialyte®).
- Eat small amounts of soft, bland foods like bananas, rice, applesauce, and toast.
- Eat foods high in protein like beef, skinless chicken or turkey, and eggs.
- Eat foods high in potassium like bananas, potatoes without the skin, avocados, and asparagus tips.
- Eat foods containing pectin like beets, applesauce without cinnamon, and peeled apples.
- Eat foods low in fiber like white bread and white rice.

Don't
- Drink alcohol, coffee or tea with caffeine, milk, or soft drinks.
- Drink very hot or cold beverages.
- Drink prune or orange juice.
- Drink grapefruit juice unless your doctor says it is okay. (Grapefruit juice can change how your medication is absorbed.)
- Drink supplements like Ensure®.
- Drink milk or eat dairy products.
- Eat spicy, greasy, or fried foods.
- Eat foods high in fiber like whole-grain bread or rice, beans, raw vegetables, seeds, popcorn, pickles, or fruit (except bananas).
- Eat foods that are very hot or very cold.

If you are going to be having radiation treatment, your doctor may suggest that you take supplements of soluble fiber (such as Metamucil®) to prevent diarrhea.

How Is Diarrhea Treated in People With Cancer?

If you are going to be having chemotherapy with drugs that are known to cause diarrhea, your doctor may give you a prescription for Imodium® (loperamide). You should start taking this medication as soon as you notice any signs of diarrhea. (Also call your doctor's office to let a member of your healthcare team know you have diarrhea.) Stop taking antidiarrheal medication once your diarrhea has subsided.

If Imodium does not work, Sandostatin® (octreotide) is another option. This medication is given by injection under the skin.

What Else Can I Do to Manage Diarrhea During Cancer Treatment?

When you have diarrhea, you need to take care of the skin around your rectum. After every bowel movement, clean your rectum with mild soap and water. Pat it dry with a soft towel. If you wish, apply a thin layer of ointment to the skin around your rectum. This can provide added protection by keeping out moisture.

If you have pain or redness in your rectum, a sitz bath may help. Sit with your buttocks and hips in warm water for 20–30 minutes. You can do this in a regular bathtub or in a special type of tub that sits over a toilet. Add salts to the water if you wish or if your doctor recommends it. Sitting in warm water allows more blood to reach the rectal area. This helps relieve pain and promotes healing. Afterward, pat the rectal area dry with a clean cotton towel.

For More Information

For additional information about diarrhea, see the following resources.

American Cancer Society

- Diarrhea: www.cancer.org/Treatment/TreatmentsandSide Effects/PhysicalSideEffects/DealingwithSymptomsat Home/caring-for-the-patient-with-cancer-at-home-diarrhea

American Society of Clinical Oncology (ASCO)

- Diarrhea—ASCO Curriculum: www.cancer.net/patient/All+ About+Cancer/Treating+Cancer/Managing+Side+Effects/ Diarrhea+-+ASCO+curriculum

Oncology Nursing Society

- The Cancer Journey: Side Effects—Diarrhea: www.thecancer journey.org/side/se-7

Hair Loss

Why Does Cancer Treatment Cause Hair Loss?

T O UNDERSTAND WHY CANCER TREATMENT OFTEN causes hair loss, it helps to know a little about cancer and about how common cancer treatments like chemotherapy and radiation work.

Cancer is caused by a rapid, out-of-control cell growth. Chemotherapy and radiation work by taking aim at cells that are multiplying rapidly. Because hair is always growing, it contains many rapidly multiplying cells. When cancer treatment damages or kills these cells, the hair falls out.

Most human hair is on the head. At any given time, more hair is growing on the head than anywhere else on the body. Following chemotherapy, hair on the head often falls out first. Body hair may fall out next, followed by eyebrow hair. Hair loss affects every patient differently; some people never lose all of their body hair.

Radiation causes hair loss only when it is given to a part of the body that is covered in hair. For example, radiation to the head causes hair loss on the treated part of the head. Radiation to a part of the body not covered in hair, such as the breast, will not cause hair loss.

Complications of cancer may also cause hair loss, for example, eating poorly or having low levels of thyroid hormone (hypothyroidism). Starting or stopping the use of birth control pills or using hormone replacement therapy may cause hair loss.

Will My Hair Grow Back?

In most cases, hair grows back within a few months after chemotherapy is over. It may start to grow back even before chemotherapy is over. Sometimes hair grows back in patches or not at all. This may happen to patients who have a bone marrow or stem cell transplant as part of their cancer treatment. It may also happen to patients who take hormonal therapies that begin or continue after chemotherapy is over (for example, tamoxifen for breast cancer). After radiation treatment, hair may not grow back in the area that was treated.

Your new hair may not look or feel the same as your old hair. For example, your new hair may be straight instead of curly, or lighter or darker in color than your old hair.

Can Hair Loss During Cancer Treatment Be Prevented?

Little research is available on how to prevent hair loss during cancer treatment. Some people have tested devices that restrict blood flow to the scalp. The thinking was that cooling the scalp in this way might prevent hair loss. Scalp cooling is still studied and used outside the United States, but the U.S. Food and Drug Administration has not approved any scalp-cooling devices to prevent hair loss caused by chemotherapy.

Some studies have shown that the drug Rogaine® (minoxidil) helped hair grow back more quickly in women treated with chemotherapy for breast or gynecologic cancer. However, some of the chemotherapy drugs used in these studies are no longer used. It is not clear whether Rogaine would have the same results in patients treated with today's chemotherapy drugs.

The following hair-care strategies may be worth trying, although no studies have shown they will prevent hair loss.

- Cut your hair short before you start chemotherapy.
- Sleep on a satin pillowcase.
- Brush your hair gently.
- Wash your hair with a gentle shampoo.
- Avoid using hair dryers, hair curlers, rollers, hairsprays, hair dye, and products that permanently curl or relax your hair.

I Just Hate the Thought of Losing My Hair. What Can I Do?

First of all, know that you are not alone. For many patients, hair loss is one of the most distressing side effects of cancer treatment. Hair can be an important part of our self-identity. You may be concerned that family members and friends will see you differently, or act differently toward you, because of your hair loss. It is normal to have these feelings.

Understanding why cancer treatment makes your hair fall out—and knowing that, in most cases, your hair will grow back—may be helpful. It may also help to look at hair loss as a sign that you are moving forward in your journey through cancer.

Planning ahead about how to deal with hair loss is another coping strategy. Many patients with cancer create new identities for themselves with wigs, hairpieces, scarves, and hats or by going bald.

If you choose to go bald, keep in mind that a bald head can get cold. On chilly days, you might want to wear a warm cap. A bald head can also get sunburned, so on sunny days be sure to wear a hat.

If you want to look about the same as you always have during your cancer treatment, choose a wig *before* you lose your hair. That way, it will be easier to get a good match with your hair color and style.

Health insurance may cover at least part of the cost of a wig if you have a prescription from your doctor.

Wearing a wig can take some getting used to. Some patients find they just do not like wearing a wig because it is too hot or too itchy.

Do I Need to Do Anything Special to Care for My Scalp?

One function of hair that we do not give much thought to is that it protects the scalp from injury. Wigs, hats, and decorations on scarves may cause scratches or blisters on your scalp. Inspect your scalp for scratches, blisters, rashes, and sunburn.

If your cancer treatment includes whole brain radiation, your doctor may give you instructions about the types of creams or lotions you should use, or not use, on your scalp.

For More Information

For additional information about hair loss, see the following resources.

American Cancer Society

- Hair Loss: www.cancer.org/Treatment/TreatmentsandSide Effects/PhysicalSideEffects/DealingwithSymptomsatHome/ caring-for-the-patient-with-cancer-at-home-hair-loss

American Society of Clinical Oncology

- Managing Side Effects—Hair Loss or Alopecia: www.cancer
  .net/patient/All+About+Cancer/Treating+Cancer/Managing
  +Side+Effects/Hair+Loss+or+Alopecia

CancerCare, Inc.

- Tips for Managing Hair Loss: www.cancercare.org/pdf/fact_
  sheets/fs_hair.pdf

Look Good … Feel Better®

- Free, nonmedical, brand-neutral, national public service
  program to help people with cancer manage their treatment
  and recovery: www.lookgoodfeelbetter.org

National Cancer Institute

- Chemotherapy and You: Support for People With Cancer—
  Side Effects and Ways to Manage Them: Hair Loss: www.cancer
  .gov/cancertopics/chemotherapy-and-you/page7

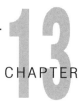

Hot Flashes

What Are Hot Flashes?

HOT FLASHES ARE BRIEF EPISODES WHEN YOUR body suddenly feels extremely hot. During a hot flash, you may start to sweat, you may feel anxious, or your heart may start to beat faster than usual. Sometimes hot flashes alternate with episodes of feeling cold. These episodes may happen several times a day or during the night. Hot flashes can disrupt sleep and interfere with your ability to carry out your usual activities. Both men and women alike can have hot flashes.

What Causes Hot Flashes in People With Cancer?

The exact cause of hot flashes is not well understood. One idea is that hot flashes occur when a part of the brain that acts as the body's thermostat is not working normally. This part of the brain usually maintains the body's temperature in a range that keeps you from getting either too hot or too cold. When the thermostat is "off kilter," body temperature may fluctuate more than normal. This results in episodes of extreme heat (hot flashes) or cold (chills).

Hot flashes may also be linked to changes in levels of sex hormones in the body. Many women get hot flashes during menopause—a time when women's bodies begin to make less of the female sex hormone estrogen. In older men, hot flashes have been linked to declining levels of the male sex hormone testosterone.

Some types of cancer can cause hot flashes. For example, women with breast cancer and men with prostate cancer have a higher likelihood of hot flashes.

Cancer treatments can cause hot flashes by altering the body's levels of sex hormones. Drugs like Nolvadex® (tamoxifen) and Femara® (letrozole) treat breast cancer by blocking estrogen's effects in the body or blocking the body's ability to make estrogen. The resulting shortage of estrogen can lead to hot flashes.

Younger women with breast cancer may be treated with combinations of chemotherapy drugs that shut down the normal menstrual cycle. This creates an "early menopause," which is often accompanied by hot flashes (see Examples of Chemotherapy Regimens for Breast Cancer That May Cause Hot Flashes).

In men, prostate cancer may be treated with drugs that block the body's ability to make testosterone. As many as three-quarters of men who are treated with these drugs have hot flashes as a side effect of treatment.

Examples of Chemotherapy Regimens for Breast Cancer That May Cause Hot Flashes
• Cyclophosphamide, methotrexate, and 5-fluorouracil • Cyclophosphamide, epirubicin, and 5-fluorouracil

Are There Tests for Hot Flashes?

It is not easy to measure hot flashes because they affect people differently. Some people find them very bothersome, and others do not. One good strategy is to keep a hot-flash diary. Record in the diary when and how often you have hot flashes, how bad they are, and other symptoms you are feeling during the hot flash.

If you are bothered by hot flashes, talk with a member of your healthcare team about them. He or she may ask questions to find out how hot flashes affect you.

Can I Do Anything to Prevent Hot Flashes?

It is not always possible to prevent hot flashes, but these tips may help make hot flashes less frequent or bothersome.
- Avoid spicy foods, caffeine, and alcohol.
- Avoid drinking very hot or very cold beverages.
- If possible, avoid going out in hot, humid weather.
- Dress so that you can quickly take off a layer of clothing if you suddenly feel too hot or add a layer if you suddenly feel too cold.
- Stopping smoking and losing extra weight may also help reduce hot flashes.

What Can Be Done to Treat Hot Flashes in People With Cancer?

Most studies of treatments for hot flashes in people with cancer have been done in women with breast cancer. Some medications used to treat depression have been found to reduce hot flashes. However, some of these medications may alter the way the body uses the drug tamoxifen and make tamoxifen less effective. If you are a woman who is taking tamoxifen and having hot flashes, ask your doctor to recommend a medication for hot flashes that will not make tamoxifen less effective (see Medications Recommended for Treating Hot Flashes in Patients With Breast Cancer).

Medications Recommended for Treating Hot Flashes in Patients With Breast Cancer		
Medication Name	**Type of Medication**	**Cautions**
Fluoxetine (Prozac®)	Antidepressant	May interfere with effectiveness of tamoxifen
Gabapentin (Neurontin®)	Anti-seizure drug	–
Paroxetine (Paxil®)	Antidepressant	May interfere with effectiveness of tamoxifen
Sertraline (Zoloft®)	Antidepressant	–
Venlafaxine (Effexor®)	Antidepressant	–

Women who have hot flashes related to menopause are often treated with low doses of the hormone estrogen or with medications that combine estrogen with another sex hormone, progesterone. Women with breast cancer, however, should not take hormonal medications. Some studies have found a higher risk of breast cancer coming back in women who took hormonal medications.

Megestrol acetate is a hormonal medication that may be effective at relieving hot flashes in both women and men. However, because some studies have suggested that it may promote tumor growth, people with cancer should not take megestrol acetate for hot flashes.

None of the studies that have been conducted so far have shown that any alternative remedies help relieve hot flashes in most people. In large studies, neither soy supplements nor the herb black cohosh reduced hot flashes any more than a place-bo ("sugar pill"). Some studies of acupuncture have shown that it helps relieve hot flashes, whereas other studies have found it had no effect. Vitamin E and hypnosis have not been studied enough to know whether they are truly helpful for treating hot flashes.

For More Information

For additional information about hot flashes, see the following resources.

American Society of Clinical Oncology (ASCO)

- Hormone Deprivation Symptoms: Men—ASCO Curriculum: www.cancer.net/patient/All+About+CancerTreating +Cancer/Managing+Side+Effects/Hormone+Deprivation +Symptoms%3A+Men+-+ASCO+curriculum
- Menopausal Symptoms: Women—ASCO Curriculum: www .cancer.net/patient/All+About+Cancer/Treating+Cancer/ Managing+Side+Effects/Menopausal+Symptoms%3A+ Women+-+ASCO+curriculum

National Cancer Institute

- Fever, Sweats, and Hot Flashes (PDQ®): www.cancer.gov/ cancertopics/pdq/supportivecare/fever/patient
- Menopausal Hormone Replacement Therapy Use and Cancer: www.cancer.gov/cancertopics/factsheet/Risk/menopaus al-hormones

Infections and Low White Blood Cell Counts

What Does It Mean if My White Blood Cell Count Is Low?

A LOW WHITE BLOOD CELL COUNT IS A COMMON side effect of some cancers and cancer treatment. When your white blood cell count is too low, you have a high risk of getting an infection. Infections can be very serious in people with cancer. If you get an infection or if your white blood cell count is very low, your chemotherapy may be delayed, and you may need to be treated in the hospital.

What Causes Low White Blood Cell Counts and Infections in People With Cancer?

White blood cells are part of your immune system, your body's built-in defense against infection. A healthy immune system contains several types of white blood cells. Each cell type plays a slightly different role in protecting you from infection. The most numerous white blood cells are called *neutrophils* (NOO-truh-fils). They are the "first responders" to viruses, bacteria, and other invaders that can cause an infection.

Similar to other white blood cells, neutrophils are made in the bone marrow. Each neutrophil takes 10–14 days to become fully mature. It then has a lifespan of hours. So the bone marrow has to keep making new neutrophils to maintain the body's supply.

As explained previously, cancer is caused by rapid, out-of-control cell growth. Chemotherapy and radiation work by taking aim at cells that are multiplying rapidly. Unfortunately, they often damage healthy cells as well as cancerous ones.

Neutrophils are always multiplying rapidly because the immune system is always making new ones. But when the immune system is damaged by chemotherapy, it stops making new neutrophils to replace the old ones. When this happens, the body quickly runs low on neutrophils.

So, a "low white blood cell count" usually means a low neutrophil count. A low neutrophil count is also called neutropenia (noo-truh-PEEN-yuh). When you have a low neutrophil count, your immune system cannot do its job of protecting you from infection as well as it normally does. When your immune system is weakened in this way, it is said to be *suppressed.*

A shortage of white blood cells can be short term (lasting less than 10 days) or long term (lasting more than 10–14 days). With many chemotherapy drugs, the number of white blood cells drops to its lowest level between 7 and 10 days after treatment. This point is called the nadir (NAY-der). Your risk of getting an infection is highest when levels of white blood cells are very low.

Are Some People With Cancer More Likely Than Others to Get a Low White Blood Cell Count?

Yes. (See Who Is Most at Risk for a Low White Blood Cell Count? and Chemotherapy Drugs More Likely to Cause a Low White Blood Cell Count.)

Who Is Most at Risk for a Low White Blood Cell Count?

- People aged 65 or older
- Women
- People who have other health problems as well as cancer (for example, diabetes; high blood pressure; and heart, kidney, or liver disease)
- People who have trouble eating a healthy diet while being treated for cancer
- People with cancers of the blood (for example, leukemia and lymphoma)
- Patients receiving their first cycle of chemotherapy
- Patients receiving high doses of chemotherapy
- Patients treated with radiation before chemotherapy or with radiation and chemotherapy at the same time
- Patients who have developed a low white blood cell count when they had chemotherapy in the past

Chemotherapy Drugs More Likely to Cause a Low White Blood Cell Count

- High-dose cyclophosphamide
- High doses of
  - Daunorubicin (Cerubidine®, Daunomycin®, DaunoXome®)
  - Doxorubicin (Adriamycin®, Doxil®)
  - Etoposide, also known as VP-16 (Etopophos®, VePesid®)
  - Idarubicin (Idamycin PFS®)
  - Mitoxantrone (Novantrone®)
  - Valrubicin (Valstar®)

What Are the Symptoms of an Infection Caused by a Low White Blood Cell Count?

When your white blood cell count is low, a fever is the most common sign of an infection. A fever means a body temperature higher than 100.4°F (38°C). Contact a member of your health-care team right away if you are running a fever. Also talk with a member of your healthcare team about how best and how often to check your temperature. It can be very dangerous for patients to have a fever of 100.4°F (38°C) or higher for a prolonged period of time without seeing a healthcare provider. This elevated temperature could be the result of a serious infection.

Other symptoms may also be a signal that you have an infection. Contact a member of your healthcare team right away if you have any of these symptoms:

- Chills or sweating
- Difficulty breathing
- Difficulty passing urine
- Diarrhea
- Stomach pain
- Discomfort in your rectum
- Tenderness in your sinuses (the air chambers in the bone behind your cheeks, eyebrows, and jaw)
- Redness or swelling at any site where a tube, or catheter, has been placed in your body.

How Do I Know if I Have a Low White Blood Cell Count?

Blood tests can tell if you have a low white blood cell count. If your white blood cell count is low or you have a fever, your doctor may order other tests to find out if you have an infection and if so, what type of infection that you have. These other tests may include a chest x-ray, lung function tests, or a computed tomography (CT) scan.

Can I Do Anything to Prevent a Low White Blood Cell Count or an Infection?

You may not be able to prevent a low white blood cell count, but you can take some simple steps to reduce your risk of getting an infection (see How to Reduce Your Risk of Getting an Infection).

How to Reduce Your Risk of Getting an Infection

- Wash your hands.
  - Always wash your hands before cooking or eating and after coughing, sneezing, or using the bathroom. Keeping hands clean is one of the simplest and most effective ways to keep an infection from spreading. Wash hands thoroughly with soap and warm water. If no soap and water is handy, use a water-free sanitizing gel.
- Avoid crowds.
  - Do your shopping and other errands during off hours and not on weekends when grocery stores and other public places are more crowded. It might be important to avoid being around other sick people, especially children.
- Get your flu shot.
  - Get a flu shot every year in the fall or early winter. If you have not had a flu shot within the past year, get one before you start chemotherapy.
  - Some people with cancer should also get a shot that protects against a type of pneumonia. Ask a member of your healthcare team if this shot is right for you.

Patients who have had a bone marrow or stem cell transplant should avoid all raw food and eat only food that has been well cooked. For other people with low white blood cell counts, however, studies have not shown that food restrictions are helpful for preventing infections.

Can Any Medications Prevent or Treat Infections Caused by a Low White Blood Cell Count?

Your doctor may want you to take a drug that speeds up the growth of white blood cells. These drugs are known as *colony-stimulating factors* (CSFs). CSFs are lab-made versions of proteins your body makes to help stimulate white blood cell growth. Studies show that patients are less likely to get a fever or very low white blood cell counts when they take CSFs during chemotherapy.

CSFs are given as shots or injections. You may get the first shot a day or two after you receive chemotherapy and every day for the next couple of weeks.

If your white blood cell count is very low or you have an infection or a fever, your doctor may prescribe antibiotics. Be sure to take the antibiotics exactly as your doctor tells you to. Even if your fever goes away, make sure you keep taking the pills for the number of days your doctor says to take them. Some patients might be admitted to a hospital for IV antibiotics if their healthcare provider determines that it is important.

For More Information

For additional information about infections, see the following resources.

American Cancer Society

- Infections in People With Cancer: www.cancer.org /Treatment/TreatmentsandSideEffects/PhysicalSide Effects/InfectionsinPeoplewithCancer/infections-in-people-with-cancer

American Society of Clinical Oncology

- Neutropenia: www.cancer.net/patient/All+About+Cancer/ Treating+Cancer/Managing+Side+Effects/Neutropenia

National Cancer Institute

- Managing Chemotherapy Side Effects: Infection: www.cancer .gov/cancertopics/chemo-side-effects/infection

Oncology Nursing Society

- The Cancer Journey: Side Effects—Prevention of Infection: www.thecancerjourney.org/side/se-9

Lymphedema

What Is Lymphedema?

LYMPHEDEMA (lim-fuh-DEMA) IS A BUILDUP OF FLUID in the body that results in swelling, usually in an arm or leg. The fluid buildup is caused by a blockage in the lymphatic (lim-FAT-ic) vessels. These vessels, which are similar to blood vessels, extend throughout your body. They carry a watery fluid called *lymph*. Lymph helps the body fight infection. It also helps remove waste products left behind by the body's infection-fighting efforts. (Think of it as the body's trash removal or plumbing system.) Lymph nodes create a chain connected to one another by the lymphatic system (think about a subway system where lymph nodes are the various stops or stations and the lymph system is the rail tracks). Lymphedema occurs when something obstructs the flow of lymph through the lymphatic vessels and causes too much fluid to build up in a limb.

What Causes Lymphedema in People With Cancer?

The most common causes of lymphedema in people with cancer are surgery to remove lymph nodes and radiation treatment.
- Surgery to remove lymph nodes: Lymph nodes are small masses of tissue in the lymphatic vessels. Clusters of lymph

nodes are found in the armpit, neck, abdomen, groin, and pelvis. Lymph nodes are often removed during cancer surgery to look for signs that the cancer has spread. Sometimes the removal of lymph nodes blocks the flow of lymph through the lymphatic vessels and causes lymphedema.

- Radiation treatment: Radiation treatment may cause lymphedema by damaging the lymphatic vessels and blocking the flow of lymphatic fluid.
- Lymphedema can also be caused by an infection or by a tumor that grows or spreads near a lymph node and blocks the lymphatic vessels.
- Lymphedema may be acute (lasting six months at most) or chronic (lasting more than six months).
- Acute lymphedema usually occurs a few days or weeks after surgery or radiation treatment. This type of lymphedema usually goes away as the body heals.
- Chronic lymphedema may occur shortly after surgery or radiation treatment or years later. This type of lymphedema can become a lifelong problem.

What Are the Symptoms of Lymphedema?

Swelling, warmth, redness, and tenderness in an arm or leg are the most common symptoms of lymphedema. You may notice that clothing or jewelry feels tight on the affected limb. You may also feel aching or heaviness in the affected limb. You may have trouble moving the limb. The skin on the affected arm or leg may become hard, thick, or pitted like orange peel.

Are There Tests for Lymphedema?

A basic test for lymphedema is to check for swelling by measuring the thickness of the arm or leg with a tape measure.

Also, the amount of fluid in a swollen limb can be measured by placing the arm or leg in a water tank and checking how much water is displaced.

Your doctor may order imaging tests such as ultrasound, computed tomography (CT) scanning, or magnetic resonance imaging (known as MRI). These tests create pictures of the lymphatic vessels that can show where the vessels are blocked. Lymphoscintigraphy (lim-foe-sin-TIG-raffee) is a special imaging test in which a radioactive substance is injected into the lymphatic vessels.

Your doctor may also run tests to rule out other causes for the swelling, such as an allergic reaction, a blood clot, heart disease, or liver or kidney failure.

Can Lymphedema Be Prevented?

These steps may help prevent lymphedema or keep it from getting worse.

- If you notice any symptoms of lymphedema, tell a member of your healthcare team right away. Lymphedema can often be cured when it is detected and treated early.
- Keep the skin on the affected arm or leg clean and dry. After bathing or showering, apply lotion to keep the skin moist. Avoid cuts, scratches, or insect bites that could cause an infection or inflammation.
- Keep the affected limb above the heart when possible.
- Keep nails clean and short. Avoid cutting the skin when trimming nails. Avoid using artificial nails.
- Avoid having needles injected into the affected arm or leg. For example, have blood drawn on the unaffected arm.
- Have your blood pressure checked on the unaffected arm.
- Avoid hot tubs, heating pads, and very hot showers to protect the affected limb from heat.

- When outdoors, use sunscreen on the affected limb. Sunburn might initiate the development of lymphedema.
- Avoid tight-fitting clothing, jewelry, or elastic bands on the affected limb.
- Be cautious when shaving the affected leg or underarm with a razor. Using an electric razor might lessen the risk of initiating lymphedema.
- Avoid carrying a heavy purse or briefcase on the affected arm.
- For lymphedema of the leg, avoid standing or sitting for long periods. When seated, avoid crossing your legs.
- Maintain a healthy body weight.
- If you have diabetes, keep blood sugar levels well controlled.

How Is Lymphedema Treated?

Manual lymph drainage (MLD) can help move lymphatic fluid from a swollen area to an unblocked area. MLD is like a gentle massage. Avoid MLD if you have open skin wounds, skin infections, or blood clots.

Compression bandaging involves wrapping the affected limb in layers of bandages. This helps move lymphatic fluid out of a swollen area and stop more fluid from building up.

Compression garments are special clothing that puts controlled pressure on parts of the arm or leg. This helps move lymphatic fluid and keep it from building up. These garments may be custom-made for a correct fit. If you have chronic lymphedema, you may need to wear a compression garment on the affected limb every day.

Lymphedema can become worse at a high altitude. If you travel by air, always wear a compression garment on the affected limb.

Exercise can be helpful for lymphedema. Stretching and contracting muscles in the affected limb can help move lymphatic fluid and reduce swelling. Always exercise with a trained therapist and bandage the limb before you exercise it.

A mechanical pump is a device connected to a sleeve that is wrapped around the arm or leg and applies pressure on and off. It is another tool for possibly moving fluid through the lymphatic vessels. Studies suggest, however, that pumps may be less helpful for lymphedema than MLD and compression garments. Pumps may also cause swelling in the area next to the sleeve. Ask your healthcare provider to help you decide which option is the best intervention for lymphedema.

Surgery may be recommended when MLD, compression, and exercise do not help. Surgery can reduce the size and weight of the affected limb. It does not, however, cure lymphedema. After surgery, you will still need to wear a compression garment to prevent fluid buildup in the affected limb.

Laser therapy is a fairly new treatment for lymphedema. A battery-powered, handheld device aims low-level laser beams at the affected limb. This may help reduce swelling and skin hardness after a mastectomy (surgery to remove a cancerous breast).

Medications have a limited role in treating lymphedema. If lymphedema is painful, your doctor may prescribe medication for the pain. An infection in a limb affected by lymphedema should be treated with antibiotics. Diuretics (drugs that reduce the amount of water in the body) may make lymphedema worse and should be avoided.

For More Information

For additional information about lymphedema, see the following resources.

American Society of Clinical Oncology (ASCO)

- Fluid in the Arms or Legs or Lymphedema—ASCO Curriculum: www.cancer.net/patient/All+About+Cancer/Treating+Cancer/Managing+Side+Effects/Fluid+in+the+Arms+or+Legs+or+Lymphedema+-+ASCO+curriculum

National Cancer Institute

- Lymphedema (PDQ®): www.cancer.gov/cancertopics/pdq/supportivecare/lymphedema/Patient/page1

National Lymphedema Network

- 18 Steps to Prevention Revised: Lymphedema Risk-Reduction Practices: www.lymphnet.org/lymphedemaFAQs/riskReduction/riskReduction.htm

Oncology Nursing Society

- The Cancer Journey: Side Effects—Swelling (Lymphedema): www.thecancerjourney.org/side/se-16

CHAPTER

Mineral and Hormone Imbalances

What Are Body Minerals, and Why Are They Important?

IMPORTANT BODY MINERALS INCLUDE CALCIUM, sodium, potassium, and magnesium. The technical term for these minerals is *electrolytes*. They play many key roles in keeping your body working normally.

To stay healthy, your body needs just the right amounts of minerals. When levels of minerals in the blood are too high or too low, many body functions can quickly get "out of whack." Abnormal levels of minerals in the blood are known as *electrolyte imbalances* (see Shedding Light on Electrolytes: What They Are, What They Do, and What Can Go Wrong).

Shedding Light on Electrolytes: What They Are, What They Do, and What Can Go Wrong			
Mineral	What It Does	Where It Is Found	What Can Go Wrong
Calcium	• Helps form and maintain healthy teeth and bones • Helps blood clot • Helps maintain a normal heartbeat	Mostly stored in the bones; a small amount is in muscle cells and the blood	Level of calcium in the blood is too low (hypocalcemia) or too high (hypercalcemia)

(Continued on next page)

(Continued)

Shedding Light on Electrolytes: What They Are, What They Do, and What Can Go Wrong			
Mineral	**What It Does**	**Where It Is Found**	**What Can Go Wrong**
Calcium *(cont.)*	• Helps muscles contract • Helps transmit nerve signals		
Sodium	• Helps the body maintain water balance • Helps muscles and nerves function properly • Helps control blood pressure	In the blood and in fluid around cells	Level of sodium in the blood is too low (hyponatremia) or too high (hypernatremia)
Potassium	• Helps build muscle • Helps the body grow normally • Helps cells and organs work properly	Mostly inside cells	Level of potassium in the blood is too low (hypokalemia) or too high (hyperkalemia)
Magnesium	• Helps the body absorb calcium • Helps maintain bones and teeth • Helps blood clot • Helps maintain a normal heartbeat • Helps transmit nerve signals	Mostly stored in the bones; a small amount is in the blood	Level of magnesium in the blood is too low (hypomagnesemia) or too high (hypermagnesemia)

How Do Mineral Levels Become Unbalanced?

Changes in the amount of fluid in the body are a common reason for mineral levels to get too high or too low. A key function of minerals, especially sodium, is to help the body maintain normal fluid levels. When you are healthy, your kidneys help keep fluid levels in balance by controlling how much fluid and minerals you excrete in urine.

Cancer treatments can upset your body's fluid balance. For example, if you have treatment side effects such as diarrhea and vomiting, your body can lose a lot of water. Some cancer treatments can affect kidney function. Damaged kidneys do not perform as well as they should at keeping fluid and mineral levels in balance.

Cancer itself can sometimes cause electrolyte imbalances. Chemotherapy and radiation treatment, as well as other kinds of medication that people with cancer may take, can also cause mineral levels in the blood to become too high or too low.

The most common mineral imbalance in people with cancer is too much calcium in the blood (hypercalcemia). Many types of cancer can cause this imbalance. Some people whose cancer has spread to the bones have a higher risk for hypercalcemia.

What Are the Symptoms of an Electrolyte Imbalance?

Many kinds of symptoms may signal an imbalance of mineral levels (see Symptoms of an Electrolyte Imbalance).

Symptoms of an Electrolyte Imbalance		
Calcium	Levels too high (hypercalcemia): • Abnormal heartbeat • Constipation • Feeling confused • Feeling tired, weak, low on energy • Pain in the stomach or side • Urinating more than normal • Vomiting	Levels too low (hypocalcemia): • Brittle nails, coarse hair, dry skin • Cramps in arms and legs • Itching • Muscle twitching • Tingling around mouth or in fingers and toes

(Continued on next page)

(Continued)

Symptoms of an Electrolyte Imbalance	
Sodium	Levels too high (hypernatremia): • Dry mouth, dry skin • Feeling restless, irritable • Feeling tired, weak, low on energy • Muscle twitching • Rapid heartbeat • Trembling, moving unsteadily, staggering	Levels too low (hyponatremia): • Feeling confused • Feeling tired, weak, low on energy • Headache • Muscle twitching • Seizures
Potassium	Levels too high (hyperkalemia): • Burning, itching, tingling in the skin • Diarrhea • Nausea, vomiting • Feeling tired, weak, low on energy • Slow heartbeat • Stomach cramps • Urinating less than normal • Weak pulse	Levels too low (hypokalemia): • Feeling confused • Feeling depressed • Feeling tired, weak, low on energy • Rapid breathing • Rapid heartbeat • Weak pulse
Magnesium	Levels too high (hypermagnesemia): • Feeling confused • Feeling weak • Nausea, vomiting • Sweating	Levels too low (hypomagnesemia): • Dizziness • Feeling confused • Feeling tired, weak, low on energy • Mood changes • Muscle cramps • Nausea, vomiting • Rapid, jerky eye movements

How Is an Electrolyte Imbalance Diagnosed?

An electrolyte imbalance is diagnosed when blood tests show that blood levels of one or more minerals are too high or too low.

Can I Do Anything to Prevent Electrolyte Imbalances?

While you are going through cancer treatment, you may not always be able to prevent imbalances of some minerals. You can take steps, though, to prevent these imbalances from becoming serious. For example,

- Talk with your healthcare team. Be sure you understand the plan to treat your cancer and the possible side effects of treatment. Learn the side effects and when to call a member of your healthcare team if you experience any of them.
- Talk with a dietitian about what foods to eat to ensure that you have the minerals your body needs. A dietitian can also help you understand how much and what kinds of fluids to drink to help keep your body in fluid balance.
- Know the symptoms of dehydration. These symptoms signal that your body is low on fluids. Talk with your healthcare team about what to do if you have any of these symptoms. (See What Are the Symptoms of Dehydration?)
- Be sure you understand how and when to take the medications or mineral supplements your doctor prescribes. (For example, some drugs and supplements should be taken when you eat. Others you should take on an empty stomach.) Do not take higher doses of medications or supplements than what your doctor prescribes.
- Keep your bones strong by walking and being as active as you can be.

What Are the Symptoms of Dehydration?

Dehydration means the body has lost too much water. Vomiting, diarrhea, drugs that increase urination, and drinking too little water can cause dehydration. These symptoms can signal dehydration:

- Dry mouth
- Dry skin
- Faintness or lightheadedness on standing up
- Feeling very thirsty
- Sweating less than usual
- Urinating less than usual.

How Are People With Cancer Treated for Electrolyte Imbalances?

The best treatment for an electrolyte imbalance depends on several things.

- Which mineral is out of balance?
- Is the problem that the level of the mineral is too high or that it is too low?
- How bad is the imbalance?

Sometimes the way to treat a mineral imbalance is to treat the cancer that is causing it. When the level of a mineral is too high, treatment usually includes giving fluids to bring the body back into fluid balance. When it is too low, treatment usually includes giving doses of the mineral to build up the body's supply. Other medications can also help get the body back into fluid balance.

When electrolyte imbalances are severe, they need to be treated in the hospital, where the imbalance can be treated and watched more closely.

What Is Antidiuretic Hormone, and How Does Cancer Affect It?

Antidiuretic (AN-tie-die-er-etik) hormone helps the kidneys control fluid levels in the body by controlling how much water you excrete in urine. It is known as ADH for short. Another name for ADH is *vasopressin.*

Remember that a key function of minerals, especially sodium, is to help the body maintain normal fluid levels. When you are healthy, your kidneys help keep fluid levels in balance by controlling how much fluid and minerals you excrete in urine.

When levels of ADH get too high, the kidneys excrete less water. This causes sodium levels to drop because the body is retaining more water. This problem is called the syndrome of inappropriate antidiuretic hormone (SIADH).

Some cancers can cause ADH levels to get too high. So can many chemotherapy drugs and other medications that people with cancer may take. (See Medications That May Cause Syndrome of Inappropriate Antidiuretic Hormone.) Nausea, a common side effect of cancer treatment, may also cause ADH levels to get too high. Pain and stress may make SIADH worse.

Medications That May Cause Syndrome of Inappropriate Antidiuretic Hormone

- Chemotherapy drugs
  - Cisplatin (Platinol®)
  - Cyclophosphamide (Cytoxan®)
  - Ifosfamide (Ifex®)
  - Melphalan (Alkeran®)
  - Vinblastine (Velban®)
  - Vincristine (Oncovin®)
- Other medications
  - Antidepressants
  - Aspirin
  - Barbiturates (drugs sometimes used to treat anxiety, insomnia, and seizures, for example phenobarbital)
  - Diabinese® (chlorpropamide, a drug used to lower blood sugar)
  - Ibuprofen (Advil®, Motrin®)
  - Morphine
  - Some diuretics ("water pills" that increase urination)
  - Tegretol® (carbamazepine, a drug used to prevent or treat seizures)

SIADH is rare in people with cancer, but when it happens it can be extremely serious (See Symptoms of Syndrome of Inappropriate Antidiuretic Hormone).

Symptoms of Syndrome of Inappropriate Antidiuretic Hormone

Contact a member of your healthcare team right away if you have any of these symptoms:
- Loss of appetite
- Loss of urine that you cannot control
- Nausea, vomiting
- Excessive thirst
- Urinating less than usual
- Unplanned weight gain.

How Is Syndrome of Inappropriate Antidiuretic Hormone Treated?

The best treatment for SIADH depends on what is causing it. If cancer is causing it, the best treatment is usually to treat the cancer. If a drug is causing it, you may need to stop taking that drug. You may also need to restrict how much fluid you drink until the body gets back into fluid balance.

What Is Tumor Lysis Syndrome?

Tumor lysis syndrome (TLS) is a rare but extremely serious type of electrolyte imbalance. When cancer cells die, they spill their contents into the bloodstream. Think of them as unwelcome, badly behaved houseguests who leave a huge mess for their host to clean up. In the case of TLS, the kidneys' job is to clean up the mess. Sometimes there is so much mess that the kidneys just cannot remove all of it, and it starts to damage the heart, lungs, and other organs. Any kind

of cancer treatment may cause TLS (see Symptoms of Tumor
Lysis Syndrome).

Symptoms of Tumor Lysis Syndrome
Contact a member of your healthcare team right away if you have any of these symptoms: • Aching in the joints or muscles • Cloudy urine • Difficulty breathing • Feeling tired, weak, low on energy • Irregular heartbeat • Nausea, vomiting.

Can Tumor Lysis Syndrome Be Prevented?

TLS can often be prevented or detected early. During your
workup, before you begin cancer treatment, your healthcare
team will assess your risk for TLS. They will carefully review your
medical history and medication use. They will do blood tests to
check your mineral levels. They will check how well your kidneys
and liver are working. They may also check your heart function.

If you are at risk for TLS, your healthcare team will take some
preventive steps before and during your cancer treatment.
These steps usually include

• Giving IV fluids to prevent dehydration.
• Giving a drug that reduces the amount of uric acid your body
  produces. (Uric acid is one of the main waste products that
  dying cancer cells leave behind.)
• Doing blood tests every six to eight hours during the first two
  or three days of your treatment. (TLS is most likely to develop on the second or third day after treatment starts.)

You may be advised to avoid certain foods, beverages, and
medications in order to protect your kidneys (see Foods,

Beverages, and Medications to Avoid if You Are at Risk for Tumor Lysis Syndrome).

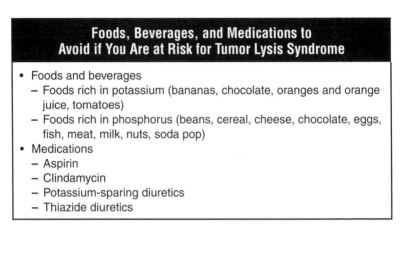

Foods, Beverages, and Medications to Avoid if You Are at Risk for Tumor Lysis Syndrome

• Foods and beverages
  – Foods rich in potassium (bananas, chocolate, oranges and orange juice, tomatoes)
  – Foods rich in phosphorus (beans, cereal, cheese, chocolate, eggs, fish, meat, milk, nuts, soda pop)
• Medications
  – Aspirin
  – Clindamycin
  – Potassium-sparing diuretics
  – Thiazide diuretics

For More Information

For additional information about mineral imbalances, see the following resources.

American Society of Clinical Oncology

• Hypercalcemia: www.cancer.net/patient/All+About+Cancer/Treating+Cancer/Managing+Side+Effects/Hypercalcemia

Cancer Consultants

• Electrolyte Imbalance: www.cancerconsultants.com/electrolyte-imbalance

National Cancer Institute

• Hypercalcemia (PDQ®): www.cancer.gov/cancertopics/pdq/supportivecare/hypercalcemia/Patient

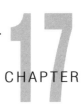

Mouth Sores

What Are Mouth Sores?

MOUTH SORES ARE SMALL ULCERS IN THE LINING of the mouth. They can be one of the most painful and frustrating side effects of cancer treatment.

Mouth sores often appear as bright red or white patches in the mouth. They may bleed or become infected. You may feel as though your mouth is very dry or your throat is hoarse. Eating or drinking (especially acidic liquids such as orange juice) may be difficult because the sores are painful. You may have trouble swallowing. Pain from mouth sores may make sleeping difficult.

What Causes People With Cancer to Have Mouth Sores?

As explained previously, cancer is caused by rapid, out-of-control cell growth. Chemotherapy and radiation work by taking aim at cells that are multiplying rapidly, like cancer cells. Unfortunately, they often damage healthy cells as well as cancerous ones. Mouth sores occur when cancer treatment damages cells in the lining of the mouth.

Radiation to the head or neck almost always causes mouth sores. The sores often appear during the second week of treatment and get worse as treatment continues. Once treatment is over, the sores gradually heal. A feeling of dryness in the mouth may continue, however, after radiation treatment is completed.

Some chemotherapy drugs are more likely than others to cause mouth sores (see Chemotherapy Drugs Likely to Cause Mouth Sores). Sores may appear two days to two weeks after chemotherapy. After a week or so the sores usually start to heal, but with the next round of chemotherapy they come back. Patients treated with bone marrow transplants have a high risk for mouth sores because of the very high doses of chemotherapy they receive.

Chemotherapy Drugs Likely to Cause Mouth Sores

- Actinomycin (dactinomycin) (Cosmegen®)
- Bleomycin (Blenoxane®)
- Busulfan (Myleran®)
- Capecitabine (Xeloda®)
- Cytosine arabinoside (Ara-C, cytarabine) (Cytosar-U®, DepoCyt®)
- Daunorubicin (daunomycin) (Cerubidine®, DaunoXome®)
- Docetaxel (Taxotere®)
- Doxorubicin (Adriamycin®)
- Doxorubicin liposomal (Doxil®)
- Etoposide VP-16 (Etopophos®, VePesid®)
- 5-fluorouracil (5-FU) (Adrucil®)
- Floxuridine (FUDF)
- Hydroxyurea (Droxia®, Hydrea®)
- Mechlorethamine (Mustargen®)
- Melphalan (Alkeran®)
- Methotrexate, high dose (Trexall®)
- Mitomycin (Mutamycin®)
- Mitoxantrone (Novantrone®)
- Paclitaxel (Taxol®)
- Procarbazine (Matulane®)
- 6-mercaptopurine (Purinethol®)
- 6-thioguanine (tioguanine) (Tabloid®)
- Thiotepa (Thioplex®)
- Vinblastine (Velban®)
- Vinorelbine (Navelbine®)

What Can Be Done to Prevent Mouth Sores in People With Cancer?

It may not be possible to completely prevent mouth sores, but you can take steps to keep them from getting worse.

- Keep your mouth clean.
- If possible, have a dental checkup before you start chemotherapy or radiation. Fixing any dental problems before you start cancer treatment may help reduce the chance of getting infected mouth sores.
- Check your mouth once a day for swelling, redness, white patches, bleeding, discomfort, or anything that "feels different." Wash your hands before examining your mouth. Stand in a strong light or use a flashlight to help you get a good look.
- Tell a member of your healthcare team right away if you notice any changes in your mouth or in how food tastes.
- Brush all the surfaces of your teeth with a soft toothbrush for 90 seconds at least twice a day. If brushing is painful, use a sponge or a piece of gauze wrapped around a finger instead of a brush.
- To prevent infection, let your toothbrush dry before storing it. Replace your toothbrush often.
- Floss your teeth at least once a day. If flossing is a new practice for you, check with your doctor or healthcare provider before initiating flossing, as there might be a concern for bleeding risk.
- Rinse your mouth four times a day with salt water, baking soda, or a mixture of the two. Use vigorous motions with the mouthwash inside the mouth.
- Avoid mouthwashes that contain alcohol.
- Do not smoke.
- Avoid foods and fluids that are hot, acidic, spicy, or coarse.

- Drink plenty of fluids (but avoid alcohol).
- Use a water-based moisturizer to keep your lips moist.

During chemotherapy with the drugs fluorouracil (5-FU) or melphalan, try sucking on ice chips. Studies show that this may keep mouth sores from getting worse. Hold the ice chips in your mouth for 5 minutes before and 30 minutes after treatment. (This tip applies *only* to treatment with 5-FU or melphalan.)

How Are Mouth Sores Treated?

In patients who are receiving a bone marrow transplant along with high-dose chemotherapy and radiation, studies have shown that the drug palifermin keeps mouth sores from getting worse and helps them heal sooner. This drug is given by injection into a vein starting three days before treatment begins and for three days after the bone marrow transplant.

Chlorhexidine (also called Peridex®, Periochip®, or Periogard®) is an antiseptic rinse often prescribed to treat infections in the mouth. Studies have shown, however, that it does not help reduce mouth sores caused by chemotherapy or radiation.

For More Information

For additional information about mouth sores, see the following resources.

American Cancer Society

- Mouth Sores: www.cancer.org/Treatment/TreatmentsandSide Effects/PhysicalSideEffects/DealingwithSymptomsatHome/ caring-for-the-patient-with-cancer-at-home-mouth-sores

American Society of Clinical Oncology (ASCO)

- Mouth Sores or Mucositis—ASCO Curriculum: www.cancer
  .net/patient/All+About+Cancer/Treating+Cancer/
  Managing+Side+Effects/Mouth+Sores+or+Mucositis
  +-+ASCO+curriculum

National Cancer Institute

- Oral Complications of Chemotherapy and Head/Neck
  Radiation (PDQ®): www.cancer.gov/cancertopics/pdq/
  supportivecare/oralcomplications/Patient/page5

Oncology Nursing Society

- The Cancer Journey: Side Effects—Mouth Irritation: www.the
  cancerjourney.org/side/se-10

Nausea and Vomiting

What Are Nausea and Vomiting?

NAUSEA IS A FEELING THAT YOU ARE GOING TO throw up. Vomiting is throwing up. They are very common side effects of cancer chemotherapy. For many people with cancer, nausea and vomiting are among the most distressing side effects of cancer treatment.

Nausea and vomiting often occur together. It is possible, however, to have nausea without vomiting or to vomit without having nausea.

Many people who have nausea and vomiting lose their appetite and then lose weight because they are not eating or drinking enough. When you have nausea or vomiting you may feel very tired. You may also feel as though you just cannot concentrate on anything.

Why Does Cancer Treatment Cause Nausea and Vomiting?

Cancer treatment sets in motion a complex chain of events in the body and brain that lead to nausea and vomiting. Chemotherapy triggers the release of a cascade of signaling chemicals, or neurotransmitters, in the body. These chemicals activate parts of the brain that control nausea and vomiting.

Acute nausea and vomiting happen within 24 hours of getting chemotherapy. Delayed nausea and vomiting happen more than 24 hours after getting chemotherapy. Delayed nausea and vomiting may last up to several days.

Some people get nausea and vomiting before chemotherapy. This is called *anticipatory nausea and vomiting*. Thinking about chemotherapy or seeing or smelling something that reminds you of chemotherapy may trigger it.

Some people with cancer are more likely than others to have nausea and vomiting with chemotherapy (see Who Is More Likely to Have Nausea and Vomiting With Chemotherapy?).

Who Is More Likely to Have Nausea and Vomiting With Chemotherapy?

- People younger than 50 years old
- Women
- People who drink less than one alcoholic drink per day before treatment
- People who have had nausea or motion sickness in the past
- Women who had a lot of morning sickness during pregnancy
- People who are anxious about getting chemotherapy
- People who take medication for anxiety or depression

Do All Chemotherapy Drugs Cause Nausea and Vomiting?

Not all chemotherapy drugs are the same when it comes to causing nausea and vomiting (see Examples of Chemotherapy Drugs That May Cause Nausea and Vomiting). Most people, however, get chemotherapy with two or more drugs. When chemotherapy drugs are combined, it is sometimes more likely they will cause nausea and vomiting.

Examples of Chemotherapy Drugs That May Cause Nausea and Vomiting

Likelihood of Causing Nausea or Vomiting	Drug
Level 1: Minimal (Less than 1 out of 10 patients are likely to have nausea or vomiting)	Bleomycin (Blenoxane®) Busulfan (Myleran®, Busulfex®) Fludarabine (Fludara®) Vinca alkaloids (for example, vinblastine [Velban®], vincristine [Oncovin®], and vinorelbine [Navelbine®])
Level 2: Low (1–3 out of 10 patients are likely to have nausea or vomiting)	Capecitabine (Xeloda®) Etoposide (VP-16; Etopophos®, VePesid®) Gemcitabine (Gemzar®) Liposomal doxorubicin (Doxil®) Methotrexate (Trexall®) Mitomycin (Mutamycin®) Mitoxantrone (Novantrone®) Taxanes (for example, docetaxel [Taxotere®] and paclitaxel [Taxol®]) Topotecan (Hycamtin®)
Level 3: Moderate (3–9 out of 10 patients are likely to have nausea or vomiting)	Carboplatin (Paraplatin®) Cyclophosphamide (dose of 1,500 mg/m^2 or lower) (Cytoxan®) Cytarabine (dose higher than 1 g/m^2) (ARA-C) Doxorubicin (Adriamycin®) Epirubicin (Ellence®) Ifosfamide (Ifex®) Irinotecan (Camptosar®) Oxaliplatin (Eloxatin®)
Level 4: High (Nearly all patients—more than 9 out of 10—are likely to have nausea or vomiting)	Carmustine (BiCNU®) Cisplatin (doses of 50 mg/m^2 or higher) (Platinol®) Cyclophosphamide (dose higher than 1,500 mg/m^2) (Cytoxan®) Dacarbazine (DTIC-Dome®) Mechlorethamine (nitrogen mustard)

How Can Nausea and Vomiting Be Prevented During Cancer Treatment?

Doctors can give a number of different medications for nausea and vomiting caused by chemotherapy. These medications are called *antiemetics.* The main goal in giving them is to prevent nausea and vomiting.

Antiemetic medications tend to work better when two or more medications are given together. Depending on what chemotherapy drugs you are given, your doctor may want you to take two or even three antiemetic medications.

Usually, you will be given your first dose of antiemetic medications before you receive your first dose of chemotherapy. Some people incorrectly only take antiemetic medications if they feel nauseated. Instead, take these medications as directed for as many days as your doctor tells you to. It is important to keep taking the medications even if you do not feel sick.

This routine of taking antiemetic medications before chemotherapy and for several days afterward will be repeated at every round of chemotherapy.

I Am Taking My Antiemetic Medications, but I Am Having Nausea and Vomiting Anyway. What Should I Do?

Antiemetic medications often do a better job of preventing acute nausea and vomiting (within 24 hours of chemotherapy) than delayed nausea and vomiting (more than 24 hours after chemotherapy). So, you may still have some nausea or vomiting several days after chemotherapy, even if you are taking the antiemetic medications your doctor has prescribed.

If you have delayed nausea or vomiting, tell a member of your healthcare team right away because dehydration is a concern in people who have prolonged nausea and vomiting.

You may need additional antiemetic medication, or a different combination of medications. People respond to antiemetic medications differently. It may take two or three attempts to find the combination of medications that works best for you.

When you go for your next doctor visit, a member of your healthcare team should ask you if you are having delayed nausea and vomiting. He or she should also check you for adverse effects such as weight loss. If no one asks you about nausea and vomiting, be sure to bring it up yourself.

What Else Can I Do to Cope With Nausea and Vomiting Caused by Chemotherapy?

In addition to taking the antiemetic medications your doctor prescribes, these steps may help you cope with nausea and vomiting during chemotherapy.

- Try acupuncture or acupressure. Some studies have shown that these complementary therapies might help reduce nausea and vomiting in people with cancer who are being treated with chemotherapy.
- Try guided imagery, music therapy, or muscle relaxation. These "mind-body" techniques may be especially helpful if you suffer from anticipatory nausea or vomiting (when you get sick just thinking about chemotherapy or when something you see or smell reminds you of it).
- See a dietitian for help finding out what foods you can eat and what foods you may want to avoid during chemotherapy.

For More Information

For additional information about nausea and vomiting, see the following resources.

American Cancer Society

• Nausea and Vomiting: www.cancer.org/Treatment/Treatments andSideEffects/PhysicalSideEffects/NauseaandVomiting/ NauseaandVomiting/index?sitearea=MBC

American Society of Clinical Oncology (ASCO)

• Nausea and Vomiting—ASCO Curriculum: www.cancer.net/ patient/All+About+Cancer/Treating+Cancer/Managing+ Side+Effects/Nausea+and+Vomiting+-+ASCO+curriculum

National Cancer Institute

• Managing Chemotherapy Side Effects: Nausea and Vomiting: www.cancer.gov/cancertopics/chemo-side-effects/nausea

Oncology Nursing Society

• The Cancer Journey: Side Effects—Nausea and Vomiting: www.thecancerjourney.org/side/se-11

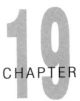

Peripheral Neuropathy

What Is Peripheral Neuropathy?

PERIPHERAL NEUROPATHY (per-IF-er-al nyoo-RAW-pah-thee), or PN, is a condition that affects the nerves that extend out from the spinal cord.

Your body's nervous system has two parts: the central nervous system and the peripheral nervous system. The central nervous system is made up of the brain and spinal cord. The peripheral nervous system is made up of all the nerves that extend out from the spinal cord to the rest of the body, including the arms, hands, legs, and feet. Damage to these nerves results in PN.

What Causes People With Cancer to Have Peripheral Neuropathy?

The peripheral nerves carry important information back and forth from the brain and spinal cord to every other part of the body. Some types of cancer and some chemotherapy drugs can damage the fibers of the peripheral nerves (see Examples of Chemotherapy Drugs That Can Cause Peripheral Neuropathy). When these nerves are damaged, they cannot do their job of carrying information back and forth as well as they normally do. This nerve damage produces the symptoms of PN.

Examples of Chemotherapy Drugs That Can Cause Peripheral Neuropathy	

• Bortezomib (Velcade®)
• Ixabepilone (Ixempra®)
• Platinum-containing agents
  – Carboplatin (Paraplatin®)
  – Cisplatin (Platinol®)
  – Oxaliplatin (Eloxatin®)
	• Taxanes
	  – Docetaxel (Taxotere®)
	  – Paclitaxel (Taxol®)
	• Thalidomide
	• Vinca alkaloids
	  – Vinblastine (Velban®)
	  – Vincristine (Oncovin®)

What Are the Symptoms of Peripheral Neuropathy?

The most common symptoms of PN are numbness and tingling in the fingers and toes. But because PN can affect nerves in almost any part of the body, it can also cause many other symptoms (see Symptoms That May Be Caused by Peripheral Neuropathy).

Unlike many cancer symptoms, the symptoms of PN are often subtle and may not be apparent to anyone except you. A few patients report PN so severe that they might have trouble walking related to the loss of feeling in their feet and toes. Members of your healthcare team may not know you are having PN symptoms unless you tell them. If you are having PN symptoms but no one asks you about them, do not keep them to yourself. Talk with a member of your healthcare team about the symptoms you are having.

Symptoms That May Be Caused by Peripheral Neuropathy
• Numbness, tingling, or burning in the fingers, hands, arms, toes, feet, and legs • Feeling that you cannot tell where your hands or feet are • Tripping, falling, or having trouble walking • Dropping things • Trouble picking up small items (such as a pin or needle)

(Continued on next page)

(Continued)

Symptoms That May Be Caused by Peripheral Neuropathy
• Trouble fastening buttons or zippers   • Changes in vision or hearing   • Weak muscles, muscle tremors   • Loss of reflexes   • Changes in responses to touch, sharp or dull pain, hot or cold temperature   • Constipation   • Urinating less than normal   • Changes in blood pressure   • Changes in sexual functioning

Are There Tests for Peripheral Neuropathy?

Some simple tests can be done in your doctor's office to find out if you have peripheral nerve damage. You may be asked to close your eyes during some of these tests. These tests include

- Tapping the knee or ankle with a reflex hammer. If your reflexes are healthy, your leg will extend or your foot will flex in response to the hammer tap.
- Placing a vibrating tuning fork against a knuckle to see if you can feel the vibrations.
- Brushing a cotton ball against the tips of your fingers or toes to see if you can feel the touch.
- Placing a sharp object (for example, the end of an open paperclip) against your hand or foot to see if you can tell that the object is sharp.

Can Peripheral Neuropathy Be Prevented or Treated?

No drugs or other treatments have yet been shown to reliably prevent or reduce PN in most people. In most patients, PN lessens or goes away after treatment is finished. In a few patients, PN remains for years after treatment, although many report that the severity decreases over time.

Techniques such as massage, low-impact exercise, whirlpool baths, and acupuncture may help reduce pain or discomfort caused by PN. In addition, try these tips for coping with PN symptoms:

- Tell a member of your healthcare team right away if you notice any symptoms that might be caused by PN.
- Take care to avoid falling.
  - Use a nonskid mat in the bathtub or shower to prevent slipping.
  - If you have trouble feeling your feet, you may find it helpful to keep your eyes on your feet as you walk. But be sure to look up often to avoid bumping into things.
  - If you feel unsteady on your feet, consider using a cane or a walker to help you keep your balance.
- Look after your feet. Inspect them regularly for injury. Wear comfortable, well-fitting shoes.
- Take care to prevent burns.
  - Lower the temperature on your hot water heater.
  - Before taking a bath or shower, test the water temperature with a thermometer.

For More Information

For additional information about PN, see the following resources.

American Cancer Society

- Peripheral Neuropathy Caused By Chemotherapy: www.cancer .org/Treatment/TreatmentsandSideEffects/PhysicalSide Effects/ChemotherapyEffects/PeripheralNeuropathy/index

American Society of Clinical Oncology

- Nervous System Side Effects: www.cancer.net/patient/All+ About+Cancer/Treating+Cancer/Managing+Side+Effects/ Nervous+System+Side+Effects

Oncology Nursing Society

- The Cancer Journey: Side Effects—Numbness or Tingling in Hands and Feet (Peripheral Neuropathy): www.thecancer journey.org/side/se-12

Problems With Thinking and Memory

Why Do I Feel Like My Brain Is in a Fog?

BOTH CANCER AND CANCER TREATMENT CAN cause problems with memory and thinking ability. These problems are often called *chemo brain* or *chemo fog*. Many people with cancer notice these problems while they are going through chemotherapy. However, people with cancer who are not undergoing chemotherapy report having similar problems (see Symptoms of Thinking and Memory Problems in People With Cancer).

Researchers have many theories about what causes problems with thinking and memory in people with cancer. However, the root causes of these problems are not well understood.

Symptoms of Thinking and Memory Problems in People With Cancer

- Memory lapses
- Short attention span, trouble focusing on a task
- Difficulty with planning or organizing
- Trouble recalling dates, events, names, or words
- Difficulty doing more than one thing at a time
- Slow thinking, taking longer than usual to finish a task
- Confusion, feelings of brain "fogginess"

Is There a Way to Prevent or Treat Problems With Thinking and Memory?

So far, doctors have not found a way to prevent thinking and memory problems in people with cancer. No drugs are approved in the United States specifically to treat these problems in people with cancer. Some people have been helped by medications for sleep disorders and attention deficit/hyperactivity disorder (commonly known as ADHD). Some women with breast cancer have been helped by therapy that teaches ways of coping with thinking and memory problems. People with other types of cancer might be helped by learning the same coping skills, but they have not been tested by research yet.

What Can I Do to Cope With Thinking and Memory Problems During My Cancer Treatment?

First of all, know that you are not imagining it. Many people with cancer report having similar problems. In most cases, thinking and memory problems during cancer treatment are temporary. Once you have completed your treatment, the feeling that your brain is in a fog should start to go away.

Many people with cancer have developed their own ways of coping with thinking and memory problems. These tips may help you, too (see Tips for Coping With Thinking and Memory Problems During Cancer Treatment).

Tips for Coping With Thinking and Memory Problems During Cancer Treatment

- Have a place for everything and put everything in its place.
  - Always keep items you use frequently in the same place so they do not get lost.

(Continued on next page)

(Continued)

Tips for Coping With Thinking and Memory Problems During Cancer Treatment

- – If you are going to need to take something out of the house with you, place it close to the door or on the doorknob.
- Get organized.
  - – Keep a to-do list. Use a grocery list when you shop.
  - – Write things down in a day planner or calendar.
  - – Use sticky notes to write reminders to yourself.
  - – Write a note to carry with you to remind yourself where you parked your car.
- Keep a journal.
  - – Look for patterns in your thinking and memory problems. Being aware of these patterns may help you find ways around them.
  - – Keep track of the problems you have and when you have them. Share these problems with a member of your healthcare team.
- Ask family members, friends, and coworkers for help.
  - – Read your journal to see where you need help.
  - – Ask family members and coworkers to take over some of your tasks.
  - – Ask friends to call to remind you of plans you have made together.
  - – Tell people around you how you are feeling. This will help them understand what you are going through.
- Work your mind.
  - – Try doing word or number puzzles to help with concentration and word-finding skills.
  - – Try doing math problems in your head, like working out how much change you will get when paying for a purchase.
- Work your body.
  - – Exercise will help you feel less tired. It can also help you sleep better. Feeling less tired and sleeping better may lessen your thinking and memory problems.
- Take good care of yourself.
  - – Use a pill box to keep track of your medications.
  - – Take notes during healthcare visits.
  - – Ask to record conversations with members of your healthcare team to help you remember what they tell you.
- Try to fix any other problems that may be making your thinking and memory problems worse.
  - – Talk to a member of your healthcare team if you are feeling sad, anxious, or tired or if you are having trouble sleeping.
  - – Have blood tests for anemia or thyroid problems.

(Continued on next page)

(Continued)

Tips for Coping With Thinking and Memory Problems During Cancer Treatment

• Try "self talk."
  – When you have a memory lapse and can feel yourself getting upset, talk to yourself to stay calm.
  – Take a deep breath and tell yourself everything is fine.
• "De-stress."
  – Try quiet activities like yoga, exercise, reading, meditation, or listening to calming music.
  – Laugh!

For More Information

For additional information about thinking and memory problems, see the following resources.

American Cancer Society

• Chemo Brain: www.cancer.org/Treatment/Treatmentsand SideEffects/PhysicalSideEffects/ChemotherapyEffects/chemo -brain?sitearea=MBC

American Society of Clinical Oncology

• Cognitive Problems: www.cancer.net/patient/All+About+ Cancer/Treating+Cancer/Managing+Side+Effects/Cognitive +Problems

Mayo Foundation for Medical Education and Research

• Chemo Brain: www.mayoclinic.com/health/chemo-brain/ DS01109

National Cancer Institute

• Managing Chemotherapy Side Effects: Memory Changes: www.cancer.gov/cancertopics/chemo-side-effects/memory

CHAPTER

Skin and Nail Changes

What Kinds of Skin and Nail Changes Can People With Cancer Experience?

SEVERAL KINDS OF SKIN AND NAIL CHANGES CAN occur as a result of some types of cancer treatment (like chemotherapy, radiation, and other specific drugs).

• You may notice a rash or dark spots on the skin or nails.

• Your skin may become very dry, or it may peel or itch.

• Fingernails or toenails may split, stop growing, change color, or become infected.

• Blood may collect under a nail.

• Sores and blisters may form on the hands and feet, especially on the palms and soles.

These changes can be painful and distressing. Sometimes, they can make it hard to walk, wear shoes, or use your hands. They can alter your appearance in ways that you may find embarrassing.

Changes such as a skin rash may appear within a week or two of starting cancer treatment. Nail changes may not appear until several weeks or months after treatment begins. The good news is that skin and nail changes go away when treatment is over.

What Causes Skin and Nail Changes in People With Cancer?

Skin and nail changes are common side effects of treatment with some cancer drugs. Many of the newer drugs attack cancer in different ways than older chemotherapy agents do. As explained earlier in this book, cancer is caused by rapid, out-of-control cell growth. Chemotherapy drugs work by taking aim at cells that are multiplying rapidly. Unfortunately, as well as killing cancer cells, chemotherapy drugs often damage healthy cells. Damage to healthy cells can cause symptoms like hair loss (see Chapter 12), low white blood cell counts (see Chapter 14), and nausea and vomiting (see Chapter 18).

Some newer cancer drugs, by contrast, take aim at specific abnormalities in cancer cells. These drugs—often called *targeted therapies*—do not damage healthy cells in the same ways that standard chemotherapy drugs do. This means that patients who take them may be spared some of the common side effects of chemotherapy. However, these drugs have their own side effects.

The "target" of many targeted therapies is epidermal growth factor receptor (EGFR). EGFRs are located on many normal epithelial tissues like skin, hair follicles, and nails, and the receptor is activated by proteins resulting in normal cell function. When EGFR is activated, it triggers cells to grow and multiply. EGFR is also found on the surfaces of cancer cells. In fact, EGFR is found at abnormally high levels on the surface of cancer cells, causing an overproduction and multiplication of cancer cells. Drugs that block or disable EGFR can help keep tumors from growing.

But there is a problem: Normal skin cells also contain EGFR. When EGFR is disabled, skin cells cannot grow normally and may have trouble retaining moisture. This can cause symptoms such as dry or peeling skin, dark spots on the skin, a rash, or nails that stop growing.

Other targeted therapies take aim at another kind of protein that helps tumors grow. In order to grow, tumors need blood vessels. Proteins called *vascular endothelial growth factor* (VEGF) and *vascular endothelial growth factor receptor* (VEGFR), as well as *platelet-derived growth factor* (PDGF) and *platelet-derived growth factor receptor* (PDGFR) help tumors to build the blood vessels they need (see Targets of Targeted Therapy: Making Sense of the Alphabet Soup). Some targeted therapies help keep tumors in check by blocking or disabling one or all of these proteins. However, when these proteins are blocked, the small blood vessels in the hands and feet can be damaged too. This damage can cause symptoms like sores on the hands and feet or blood under the nails.

Targets of Targeted Therapy: Making Sense of the Alphabet Soup	
EGFR	Epidermal growth factor receptor: protein that signals cells to grow and divide. Blocking or disabling it can help keep tumors from growing.
PDGF PDGFR	Platelet-derived growth factor and platelet-derived growth factor receptor: proteins that help tumors to build blood vessels. Blocking or disabling them can help keep tumors in check.
VEGF VEGFR	Vascular endothelial growth factor and vascular endothelial growth factor receptor: similar to PDGF/PDGFR, proteins that help tumors build blood vessels. Blocking or disabling them can help keep tumors in check.

Some other drugs used in cancer treatment can also damage skin cells, causing some of the same skin and nail changes seen with targeted therapies (see Examples of Cancer Drugs That Can Cause Skin and Nail Changes).

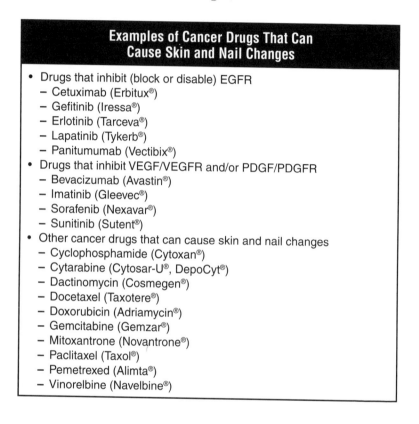

Examples of Cancer Drugs That Can Cause Skin and Nail Changes

- Drugs that inhibit (block or disable) EGFR
  - Cetuximab (Erbitux®)
  - Gefitinib (Iressa®)
  - Erlotinib (Tarceva®)
  - Lapatinib (Tykerb®)
  - Panitumumab (Vectibix®)
- Drugs that inhibit VEGF/VEGFR and/or PDGF/PDGFR
  - Bevacizumab (Avastin®)
  - Imatinib (Gleevec®)
  - Sorafenib (Nexavar®)
  - Sunitinib (Sutent®)
- Other cancer drugs that can cause skin and nail changes
  - Cyclophosphamide (Cytoxan®)
  - Cytarabine (Cytosar-U®, DepoCyt®)
  - Dactinomycin (Cosmegen®)
  - Docetaxel (Taxotere®)
  - Doxorubicin (Adriamycin®)
  - Gemcitabine (Gemzar®)
  - Mitoxantrone (Novantrone®)
  - Paclitaxel (Taxol®)
  - Pemetrexed (Alimta®)
  - Vinorelbine (Navelbine®)

Can Skin and Nail Changes Be Prevented or Treated in People With Cancer?

It is not always possible to prevent skin and nail changes. However, you can take steps that may keep skin and nail changes from becoming serious.

- Avoid skin products that contain alcohol or perfume. These substances can irritate or dry the skin.
- Clean your skin with a mild, moisturizing liquid soap.

- Use moisturizing lotion on your hands, feet, and nails. The thicker the lotion, the more it will soften and smooth your skin.
- If you have a skin rash, stay out of the sun as much as possible. When you go outdoors, always wear sunscreen with a sun protection factor (SPF) of at least 15.
- Use makeup to cover skin blemishes on your face. Ask a member of your healthcare team which kinds of makeup will not make skin blemishes worse.
- Try not to bite your nails or cuticles (the skin around your nails).
- Avoid wearing tight shoes.
- If you get your nails done at a nail salon, make sure the manicurist uses sterile equipment.

With some targeted drugs that block or disable EGFR, getting a skin rash may be a sign that your treatment is working. Knowing this may help you put up with the rash even though it may be itchy or ugly. Think about how bad a rash you can tolerate if it means your treatment will be successful. **Most importantly, do not stop taking your targeted therapy without talking to a member of your healthcare team.**

You can also talk with a member of your healthcare team if you are having a hard time dealing with skin and nail changes that alter your appearance. Consider joining a support group. It is often helpful to share experiences with other people who are facing similar challenges.

Skin blemishes that itch can be treated with antihistamines (medicines for allergies and colds). Skin infections can be treated with antibiotics. If your doctor prescribes medicine for a skin problem, be sure to take it exactly as directed. Even if your skin looks or feels better, keep taking the medication for the number of days your doctor tells you to take it.

For More Information

For additional information about skin and nail changes, see the following resources.

American Cancer Society

- Skin Changes Caused by Targeted Therapies: www.cancer .org/Treatment/TreatmentsandSideEffects/PhysicalSide Effects/ChemotherapyEffects/skin-changes-caused-by -targeted-therapies

American Society of Clinical Oncology

- Skin Reactions to Targeted Therapies: www.cancer.net/ patient/All+About+Cancer/Treating+Cancer/Managing+ Side+Effects/Skin+Reactions+to+Targeted+Therapies

Look Good ... Feel Better®

- Free, nonmedical, brand-neutral, national public service program to help people with cancer manage their treatment and recovery: www.lookgoodfeelbetter.org

National Cancer Institute

- Managing Chemotherapy Side Effects: Skin and Nail Changes: www.cancer.gov/cancertopics/coping/chemo-side-effects/ skin-and-nail

Sleep Problems

What Kind of Sleep Problems Can Be Caused by Cancer or Cancer Treatment?

ALL OF US NEED TO SLEEP. WHEN YOU ARE GOING through cancer treatment, you need your rest more than ever. However, as many as half of people with cancer sometimes have a hard time getting a good night's rest. Sleep problems caused by cancer treatment may include

- Having trouble falling asleep
- Waking up frequently during the night
- Waking up very early and having trouble going back to sleep
- Not feeling rested after a night's sleep.

If you are not sleeping well at night, chances are you will feel tired during the day. It is harder to go about your usual daytime activities when you feel tired. You may try to catch up on sleep by taking daytime naps. Too much napping during the day, however, can make it even harder to sleep well at night.

What Causes People With Cancer to Have Problems Sleeping?

Most people have a "body clock" that follows a roughly 24-hour daily cycle. Individuals' sleep-wake cycles vary—for some people, "early to bed and early to rise" comes naturally, whereas others prefer getting up and going to bed later. Hormones and other substances in the body regulate the sleep-wake cycle. Cancer and its treatment can change the levels of these substances in ways that disrupt your normal sleep-wake cycle.

Other cancer symptoms also can interfere with sleeping. People with cancer who have trouble sleeping often have other symptoms as well, such as anxiety (see Chapter 2), pain (see Chapter 6), fatigue (see Chapter 7), depression (see Chapter 10), and mouth sores (Chapter 17).

What Can I Do if I Am Having Trouble Sleeping?

These tips may help you sleep better while you are being treated for cancer.

- Do not suffer in silence. Talk with a member of your health-care team if you are not sleeping well.
- Try to go to bed and get up at about the same time every day. Having a regular schedule can train your body to know when it is time to sleep and time to wake up.
- If you cannot fall asleep, get out of bed and go to another room. Go back to bed when you feel sleepy.
- Use the bedroom for sleep and sex only. Do not watch TV or movies or surf the Internet while you are in bed.
- Keep the bedroom cool. Use light covers on the bed. It may be harder to sleep when the room or the bed is too warm.
- Avoid daytime napping. If you really need to take a nap, keep it to no more than 45 minutes.
- Within two hours before going to bed, relax by taking a warm bath or shower, reading, or listening to music.

- Avoid caffeine and alcohol in the afternoon and evening. These substances can stimulate the brain and disrupt sleep.
- Finish your evening meal three hours before going to bed. Do not go to bed hungry.
- Get regular exercise. For example, go for a 20- or 30-minute walk four or five times a week. If you can, also do strength-training exercises to keep your muscles strong. Do your exercise at least three hours before bedtime.
- Try different relaxation techniques to see which ones are most helpful for reducing stress. For example, try yoga, meditation, or massage. Try contracting and then relaxing all your muscles, from head to toe, one at a time. Try focusing on your breathing: listen to your breath coming in and going out and feel your chest rising and falling as you breathe.
- Write down your thoughts and feelings about your illness and treatment in a journal. This may make it easier to "turn off" when you go to bed.

Can I Take Medication to Help Me Sleep?

Various medications may help with sleep. None have been studied to find out how well they work in people with cancer. Most sleep aids are intended to be used only for a short time. Some sleep medications can cause daytime sleepiness. Others may help you to fall asleep but not to stay asleep all night.

Talk with your healthcare team before using any herbal products to help you sleep. Some of these products may interfere with cancer treatment and make it less effective. Be sure to tell a member of your healthcare team if you are taking any herbal sleep remedies.

For More Information

For additional information about sleep problems, see the following resources.

American Cancer Society

- Sleep Problems: www.cancer.org/Treatment/Treatments andSideEffects/PhysicalSideEffects/DealingwithSymptoms atHome/caring-for-the-patient-with-cancer-at-home-sleep-problems

American Society of Clinical Oncology

- Strategies for a Better Night's Sleep: www.cancer.net/patient/ All+About+Cancer/Cancer.Net+Features/Quality+of+Life/ Strategies+for+a+Better+Night%27s+Sleep

National Cancer Institute

- Sleep Disorders (PDQ®): www.cancer.gov/cancertopics/ pdq/supportivecare/sleepdisorders/Patient/page2

Oncology Nursing Society

- The Cancer Journey: Side Effects—Sleep Disturbances: www .thecancerjourney.org/side/se-15